D0472805

Remediation and Management of Low Vision

Remediation and Management of Low Vision

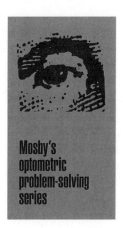

Mosby's optometric problem-solving series

Edited by

Roy G. Cole
OD, FAAO

Diplomate in Low Vision
Professor, Chief Low Vision Service
State University of New York
State College of Optometry, New York, New York

Bruce P. Rosenthal
OD, FAAO

Diplomate in Low Vision
Chief Low Vision Programs
The Lighthouse Inc., New York, New York;
Distinguished Professor, State University of New York
State College of Optometry, New York, New York

Series Editor

Richard London
MA, OD, FAAO

Diplomate, Binocular Vision and Perception
Pediatric and Rehabilitative Optometry
Oakland, California

with 54 illustrations

Mosby

St. Louis Baltimore Boston Carlsbad Chicago Naples New York Philadelphia Portland
London Madrid Mexico City Singapore Sydney Tokyo Toronto Wiesbaden

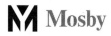 Braille Institute Library Services

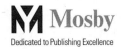
Mosby

Dedicated to Publishing Excellence

A Times Mirror Company

Executive Editor: Martha Sasser
Associate Developmental Editor: Kellie White
Project Manager: John Rogers
Series Design: Jeanne Wolfgeher
Design Coordinator: Renée Duenow
Manufacturing Supervisor: Linda Ierardi
Editing and Production: Carlisle Publishers Services

Copyright © 1996 by Mosby–Year Book, Inc.

All rights reserved. No part of this publication may be reproduced, stored in a retrieval system, or transmitted, in any form or by any means, electronic, mechanical, photocopying, recording, or otherwise, without prior written permission from the publisher.

Permission to photocopy or reproduce solely for internal or personal use is permitted for libraries or other users registered with the Copyright Clearance Center, provided that the base fee of $4.00 per chapter plus $.10 per page is paid directly to the Copyright Clearance Center, 27 Congress Street, Salem, MA 01970. This consent does not extend to other kinds of copying, such as copying for general distribution, for advertising or promotional purposes, for creating new collected works, or for resale.

Printed in the United States of America
Composition by Carlisle Communications, Ltd.
Printing/binding by Maple-Vail Book Manufacturing Group

Mosby–Year Book, Inc.
11830 Westline Industrial Drive
St. Louis, Missouri 63146

International Standard Book Number 0-8151-5204-3

95 96 97 98 99 / 9 8 7 6 5 4 3 2 1

Braille Institute Library Services

Contributors

Aries Arditi, PhD
Director, Vision Research
The Lighthouse Inc.
New York, New York

Jay M. Cohen, OD, FAAO
Associate Professor
Diplomate in Low Vision
State University of New York
State College of Optometry
New York, New York

Roy G. Cole, OD, FAAO
Professor
Diplomate in Low Vision
Chief Low Vision Service
State University of New York
State College of Optometry
New York, New York

Gregory L. Goodrich, PhD
Diplomate in Low Vision
Research Psychologist
Psychology Service and Western Blind
   Rehabilitation Center
U.S. Department of Veterans Affairs
   Medical Center
Palo Alto, California;
Assistant Clinical Professor
School of Optometry
University of California
Berkeley, California

Kent Higgins, PhD
Research Investigator
The Lighthouse Inc.
New York, New York

Wayne W. Hoeft, OD, FAAO
Clinical Professor
The Southern California College
   of Optometry
Fullerton, California;
Director of Low Vision Residencies
The Santa Monica Center for the Partially
   Sighted
Santa Monica, California;
Private Low Vision Practice
Burbank, California

Clare M. Hood, RN, MA
The Lighthouse Inc.
New York, New York

Alan L. Innes, OD, FAAO
Associate Professor
State University of New York
State College of Optometry
New York, New York

John E. Musick, OD, FAAO
Diplomate in Low Vision
Clinical Director of Low Vision
   Rehabilitation Services
Lexington, Kentucky

William O'Connell, OD, FAAO
Diplomate in Low Vision
Assistant Clinical Professor
State University of New York
State College of Optometry
New York, New York

Gary E. Oliver, OD
Associate Professor
State University of New York
State College of Optometry
New York, New York

Bruce P. Rosenthal, OD, FAAO
Diplomate in Low Vision
Chief Low Vision Programs
The Lighthouse Inc.
New York, New York;
Distinguished Professor
State University of New York
State College of Optometry
New York, New York;
Ajunct Professor
Mt. Sinai Hospital, New York
New York, New York

Theresa Sacco, MA
Computer Access Training Specialist
Western Blind Rehabilitation Center
U.S. Department of Veterans Affairs
    Medical Center
Palo Alto, California

Karen R. Seidman, MPA
The Lighthouse Inc.
New York, New York

Brendal Waiss, OD, FAAO
Assistant Clinical Professor
State University of New York
State College of Optometry
New York, New York

Douglas R. Williams, OD, FAAO
Diplomate in Low Vision
Huntington Beach, California;
Assistant Clinical Professor
Southern California College
    of Optometry
Fullerton, California

To our wives
Carol and Susan
and children
Jason, Matthew, and Daniel
and Jason, Kerrin, and Andrew

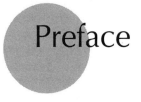

Preface

The original intent of the authors was to produce a single volume on the functional aspects of low vision care that could be included in Mosby's Optometric Problem-Solving Series. However, the body of knowledge in low vision has expanded so rapidly that functional assessment rapidly filled the first volume. A second volume was needed to deal with remediation and management considerations. This volume is therefore a companion volume to *Functional Assessment of Low Vision* (Rosenthal and Cole) published by Mosby–Year Book, Inc.

Both texts place a heavy emphasis on visual function, whether it is evaluation or remediation. The authors' intent is therefore to explore ways of making advantageous use of the residual vision.

We hope these volumes will stimulate an interest and involvement in the rapidly expanding field of low vision rehabilitation not only in the United States but throughout the world.

Acknowledgments

To Kellie White for all the initial work in laying the foundation for this book.

To Amy Dubin for all the time and effort expended in bringing everything together.

Again a special thanks to Karen Seidman for all her help in the preparation and proofreading of the chapters.

To the authors, without whose help this book could never have been written.

Roy G. Cole
Bruce P. Rosenthal

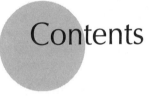

Contents

Remediation
and
Management
of Low Vision

1

Visual Field Remediation

Jay M. Cohen
Brendal Waiss

Key Terms

visual field defect	minifiers	Fresnel prism
prism	reverse telescope	head trauma
mirrors	hemianopia	

The purpose of this chapter is to introduce the reader to the concepts needed for the clinical management of patients with visual field defects. The content is based on our experiences and includes our preferred techniques. Other approaches to the problem exist and a more comprehensive overview of existing techniques has previously been published.[1] It is understood that optometric intervention cannot be done in isolation and presupposes that appropriate referral for assessments by other disciplines such as orientation and mobility, and occupational therapy just to name two, has been made.

Clinically we find that each year there is an increase in the number of patients with general visual impairment and more specifically with visual impairment secondary to compromised visual fields. This is probably due to the improved survival rates of stroke/head trauma patients, or perhaps due to the fact that patients who are diagnosed with diseases causing field problems are now coming to low vision clinicians with the expectation that help may be available for them. Unfortunately, many practitioners' first reaction to patients requiring field remediation is that there are few successful treatment options available to them. On the contrary, depending on the creative abilities of the practitioner and the willingness of the patient to explore these options, there can be successful outcomes to many of these cases.

General Considerations

Problems related to visual field loss are manifested only when two specific conditions exist: (1) the stimulus of interest, a target of active search, falls in an area of field loss and (2) the field loss is bilateral.

The first condition explains why many patients fail to report functional difficulties despite rather significant field losses and is the rationale behind many of the environmental modification strategies used in therapy. Simply put, if a stimulus falls inside the scotoma and is not being sought, then its existence is not known and the patient is unaware of the field defect. Likewise, if a stimulus falls outside of the scotoma, it will be seen and the patient will again be unaware of a defect.

The second condition explains why patients with visual field problems must suffer from either advanced bilateral eye disease or postchiasmal neurological insult. Few other pathologies will cause the bilateral symmetrical damage necessary to affect corresponding visual loci. If the field loss is monocular, then the target will be seen by the intact field of the fellow eye.

Visual field defects can be classified into two broad categories: (1) hemianopic or sector defects and (2) overall constriction. Hemianopic defects are cerebral in origin and are generally acquired after head trauma or stroke while overall constrictions are more likely caused by tapetoretinal degeneration or bilateral glaucoma and optic nerve disease.

In the case of patients with hemianopic visual field defects, we prefer to see the patients early on in the disease process so that they can begin rehabilitation and avoid the development of inappropriate adaptive behaviors. However, in the case of diseases which produce an overall constriction in field the opposite is true. The larger the remaining field, the less it impacts on mobility and daily living skills, and the less likely the patient will need enhancement of the field. By the time the patient has significant loss, the challenge is greater, but the patient should be more responsive to the various options that can be tried.

Head Trauma Induced Field Loss

Time is an important aspect when attempting field remediation on the head trauma patient. While relatively early intervention is important, head trauma patients need time to recover whatever field they are going to recover naturally. They also often need time to physically recover and mentally readapt to their new status. At some point, when the patient is stable, he is ready to begin the rehabilitative process.

A careful evaluation of oculomotor skills and cognitive status is crucial in developing a treatment plan because of the critical role of both eye and head scanning behavior in compensating for visual field loss. Head trauma patients frequently exhibit varying degrees of hemispatial neglect, an important factor influencing the choice of the best treatment modality for the field defect. Every patient should be screened for neglect by functional observation and performance tests.

Treatment of Hemifield or Sector Loss

Treatment modes incorporate elements of vision training, and optical and nonoptical techniques. Vision training develops smooth and efficient eye movements, systematic head and/or eye scanning patterns, and improved visual-spatial and body awareness. Optical techniques utilize devices, primarily prisms and mirrors, which shift incoming information from the nonfunctioning area of the field to the seeing part. Nonoptical methods include cognitive training and environmental modifications to help patients remain aware of their field limitations and to adjust for them appropriately.

The strategy behind the treatment of hemianopsia is simple even though the implementation of the remediative measures is anything but simple. The goal is to take visual information present in the nonseeing portion of the field and transfer it for processing by the functioning area of the field. Ideally, this should be done in a way which is cosmetically acceptable and which simultaneously presents an image from both fields without distorting the visual image or interfering with the visual input to the nonaffected field. In practice, this theoretical ideal does not exist, forcing the doctor and patient to compromise on one of the far from perfect alternatives.

CLINICAL PEARL

The strategy behind the treatment of hemianopsia is to take visual information present in the nonseeing portion of the field and transfer it for processing in the functioning area of the field.

Optically two categories of devices can help compensate for sector defects: mirrors and prisms.

Mirrors

Mirrors in their various forms come closest to meeting the criteria of providing simultaneous large angle compensation for sector field defects. A mirror is mounted nasally on the spectacles on the same side as the field defect (Figure 1-1). Information from the non-seen area is reflected onto the functioning area of the retina. The larger the mirror, the larger the area of coverage. Information is provided via direct reflection into the eye and by the mirror's presence as a side view mirror into which a patient can gaze to scan the field (analogous to the use of side view mirrors when driving).

Placement of the mirror provides the doctor with a great deal of control over the visual parameters. The more central the placement on the carrier lens, the greater the area of simultaneous overlap of the fields; the more nasal the placement, the greater is the dependency on the side view scanning action. The smaller the angle between the mirror and the spectacle plane, the more peripheral is the area of incoming information; the larger the angle, the more forward is that

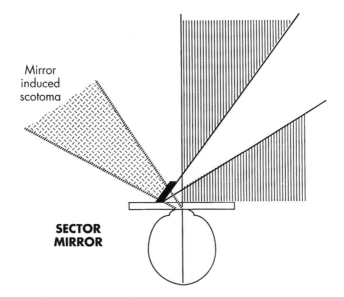

Mirror
induced
scotoma

**SECTOR
MIRROR**

FIGURE 1-1 Schematic of sector mirror. The shaded area represents the scotoma or non-seen area and the clear area represents seen information. Although the area "seen" by the mirror is physically on the right, it is preceived on the left, in the area of scotoma created by the mirror.

area. Theoretically when the mirror is perpendicular to the spectacle plane, the patient should see the straight ahead central field. When the mirror is parallel to the spectacle plane, the area behind the patient is seen. The angle adjustment capability of a mirror is one of its major advantages, as it allows the patient to choose which area of the missing field receives primary compensation. One interesting patient, a percussionist by profession, was required to alternate her attention between four widely spaced instruments. A mirror provided her with the freedom to easily locate her instruments over a large peripheral area.

Of course mirrors are no panacea for field defects. They occlude the area of functioning retina of the eye over which they are placed, thereby limiting their usefulness to binocular patients only. This problem can be partially solved by the use of semireflecting mirrors for monocular patients, although the faintly reflected image of these mirrors is difficult for many patients to appreciate[2,3] (Figure 1-2). The lab work must also be of the highest caliber as not only is the positioning crucial but the area to be silvered must have the darkest tint to produce the best mirror effect.

Dealing with the reversed image and the exaggerated movement of the image is a problem for many patients. The image is seen on the side opposite to its actual location and the patient must reproject it to the correct side in order to successfully utilize the information.

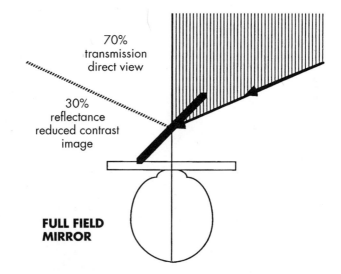

70%
transmission
direct view

30%
reflectance
reduced contrast
image

**FULL FIELD
MIRROR**

FIGURE 1-2 Schematic of a semireflecting/semisilvered full field mirror. The patient sees the low contrast reflected image superimposed over the higher contrast real world view.

Patients with neglect are incapable of this reprojection and generally are poor candidates for mirrors. On one clinical trial using a mirror on a patient with right hemianopia and neglect, every doorway on the right side of a hallway was correctly identified; however, the patient persisted in perceiving the doorway as being on the left side of the hallway, making the increased peripheral awareness of little value in a real world situation.

The biggest impediment to the use of mirrors, though, is the cosmetic factor. Most patients strongly object to the physical appearance of the mirror which projects forward from the spectacle plane. Although we have had some success using small plane mirrors mounted behind the lens, a measure which dramatically improves the cosmesis of the appliance, the patient must sacrifice a large portion of the field enhancement potential as compared to the standard anteriorly placed mirror[4] (Figure 1-3). Any time a mirror is fitted behind the lens, one must take extreme care to make sure that the mirror clears the cornea for safety and clears the eyelashes for patient comfort. One would have to caution the patient regarding safety because the mirror could theoretically make contact with the eye if there was a severe blow to that area.

Convex mirrors are devices whose potential is yet to be fully explored. They could conceivably decrease the required mirror size without adversely affecting the size of the enhanced field. The disadvantage of convex mirrors is that the image is located at a finite distance from the eye and the patient must be capable of accommodating to maintain image clarity.

Clinical management of mirrors. For clinical trials of mirrors, we prefer to use the clip-on mirror from Jardon Institute[5] (Figure 1-4). It consists of a small dental mirror soldered to a padded tie clip. It is

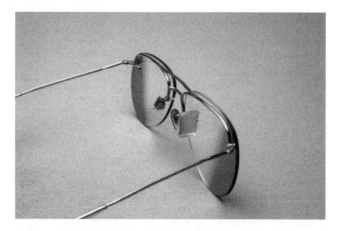

FIGURE 1-3 Behind the lens mounted mirror is a cosmetic alternative to larger anterior mounted mirrors.

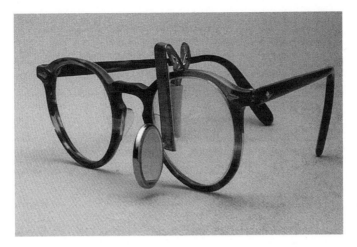

FIGURE 1-4 Clip-on mirror placement for a homonymous field defect.

available in either a right or left orientation. It is inexpensive and provides complete flexibility as to placement on the lens and some limited flexibility as to the angle of the mirror's tilt. Patients also have the option of when they choose to use the mirror since it is easily removed when desired.

Initially the patient sits comfortably in the exam chair viewing a straight ahead distance target. The mirror is positioned over the lens until the patient is aware of the reflected field. The patient is instructed in the significance of the image and taught the techniques of locating objects in the mirror and turning the eye when necessary to locate the objects in real space. The mirror is then adjusted until the best subjective placement is achieved. Finally the patient is permitted to walk around the room and hallway wearing the mirror and the position is finely tuned to produce the maximum beneficial effect. If the device is deemed safe and beneficial in the hands of the patient, he should be shown how to position the mirror and it should be loaned to the patient for a minimum one week home trial.

At follow-up, if the patient finds the mirror to be useful, it can be dispensed to the patient. A permanently mounted mirror can be fabricated by some custom optical shops but the cost is significantly higher and most of the patient's control over the position adjustment is now lost.

Prisms

Prisms are a second type of optical system used for enhancement of visual fields in the cases of sector or hemifield loss. Prisms shift the visual image toward the apex of the prism (Figure 1-5). The linear displacement is dependent on the power of the prism and the distance from the object. The intention is to shift objects within the nonseen

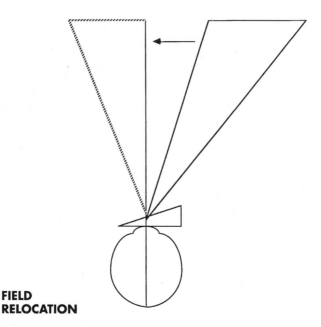

FIELD
RELOCATION

FIGURE 1-5 Schematic of overall prism relocation of a hemifield. The image is shifted to the apex of the prism.

field toward and into the seeing area of field. As one of the few ironclad clinical rules, the prism base is always placed with the base toward the field defect.

CLINICAL PEARL

The prism base is always placed with the base toward the field defect.

One point that must be strongly emphasized is that visual field defects and prism base placement correspond to the patient's, and not the doctor's, frame of reference. Thus a right hemianopia with prism base-right refers to field loss on the patient's right and to the left of the doctor facing the patient. On more than one occasion we have seen an unhappy patient, who through either doctor or optician error, was wearing prism base opposite to his needs. It is helpful when writing the prescription to avoid confusion by using base-in and base-out rather than base-right or base-left. Thus base-right would be written as base-out OD and base-in OS, whereas base-left would be written as base-in OD and base-out OS.

CLINICAL PEARL

It is helpful when writing the prescription to avoid confusion by using base-in and base-out rather than base-right or base-left. Thus base-right would be written as base-out OD and base-in OS, whereas base-left would be written as base-in OD and base-out OS.

There are two ways of utilizing prism in the spectacles of hemianopes: full field and partial prisms.

Full field prism

Full field prism offers the most cosmetically acceptable means of enhancing the visual fields and it is the only approach that is useful for both distance and near tasks. Because it affords the patient an uninterrupted field, it provides the most natural viewing conditions. Theoretically the prism is placed binocularly in the spectacle lenses and shifts the entire field away from the scotoma (Figure 1-6). The

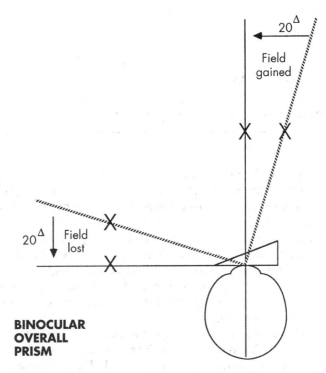

20^Δ

Field gained

20^Δ Field lost

**BINOCULAR
OVERALL
PRISM**

FIGURE 1-6 Schematic of binocular overall prism. Depicts the amount of visual field gained versus amount of visual field lost.

prism must be used binocularly to avoid inducing diplopia. Patient involvement is somewhat passive and this technique can work well with cases of neglect and cognitive impairment. Aside from the effect on the visual field, this technique can favorably alter posture and reduce compensatory body skews commonly seen after head trauma or stroke.[6]

Cosmesis and comfort of the device can influence patient acceptance. Therefore selection of an appropriate frame is important for minimizing lens thickness and weight. The key factors are selecting a frame whose distance between centers (DBC) is as close as possible to the patient pupillary distance (PD) and selecting a shape which is as small and round as possible. Plastic frames are generally better able to conceal the thick lens edge and hold the lenses more securely than metal frames. The bottom line, though, is to pick a frame with which the patient is happy in order to ensure compliance. The patient should be forewarned of the weight and possible chromatic aberrations in the final prescription. In order to decrease some of the lens thickness and to avoid some of the extra charges involved in grinding in lens prism, it is important to direct the lab to produce the lens with a combination of grinding in the prism and with prism produced by decentration if the lens power merits it. Selection of high index lens material and antireflective coating can also enhance the appearance of the finished product.

CLINICAL PEARL

Selection of high index lens material and antireflective coating can also enhance the appearance of the finished product.

Although many doctors use Fresnel prisms for this application, we much prefer using ground-in prism. In our experience binocular Fresnel prism is almost universally rejected by patients because of the decreased visual resolution inherent in its optics. Even for short term trial we avoid its use, as it causes many patients to reject the benefits of prism despite our assurances that vision will be clear with the final product. Bernell markets a prism training goggle which is available in a wide range of prism powers and can be worn alone or over glasses. This goggle is cosmetically tolerable and makes an ideal loaner and testing device (Figure 1-7).

The downside of using ground-in prism is that the practical upper limit of usable power is 15 to 20 prism diopters as compared to the 35 to 40 prism diopters obtainable with Fresnel prisms. However, for most patients the prescribed power is close to 10 prism diopters, so it is rarely necessary to compromise power for optical quality.

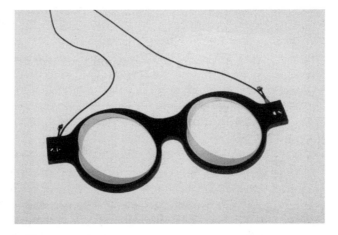

FIGURE 1-7 Rotatable prism goggles available as a stock item.

Clinical management of full field prism. As the patient fixates a distance target, 6 to 8 prism diopters of prism with the bases yoked in the direction of the field loss, is placed in front of the patient's eyes. The patient is asked to report on any subjective changes in the appearance of the field and to quantify the amount of visual field shift or increase. The patient is also observed for any postural or behavioral changes. Asking direct questions about objects in the environment should allow most patients to become cognizant of the improved awareness with prism. The power of the prism is changed in 2 to 4 prism diopters steps in both directions from the starting amount until the patient reaches the preferred lens. This prism power is then used as the starting point for determining the best lens for mobile conditions. The patient is observed walking with the prism and reports on the experience. The prism power is again modified until the best lens is found. Some patients do well under stationary conditions but have difficulty dealing with spatial distortion under dynamic use. The best lens therefore is determined based on patient comfort and performance.

One of the truly rewarding experiences working with hemianopic patients is observing the transformation in mobility skills that occurs with many of them while wearing prisms. The field defect frequently causes patients to drift away from the side with the deficit and the patient often ends up "hugging" the wall. The prism restores a sense of centeredness in many patients and permits them to ambulate with reduced drift and away from the wall.

The last area to investigate is near point performance. The patient is seated at a desk and asked to perform a series of activities such as reading, locating objects, and pencil and paper tasks. Each task is done with and without varying amounts of prism until the most appropriate power is found. In all the conditions you should try to find the weakest power the patient will accept without sacrificing performance.

At this time a decision must be made about whether to prescribe the prism or not. The decision rests on a number of factors including the perceived and/or measured benefits and the range of activities the patient wishes to perform. Multiple pairs of spectacles may be necessary if, for example, significantly different amounts of prism were found to be optimal for stationary and nonstationary tasks and if the patient requires a different spectacle prescription for distance and near.

After any prism prescription is dispensed careful follow-up is required. The patient should be warned of the possible distortions and should be given a wearing schedule. The decision as to whether the glasses should be worn intermittently or full time is based on an individual basis and patient need. Familiarization-type exercises or tasks might also be recommended to the patient to help during this adaptation period. Long term follow-up care determines the continued need for the prism. Many patients adapt to the prism over the course of months to years until they can perform just as well without the prism, allowing it to be dropped from any future prescriptions.

Partial prism

As compared to full field prism, partial prism uses an entirely different stratagem in compensating for field loss. Its primary action is to reduce the amplitude of the scanning eye movements into the blind field, rather than to increase awareness of the field (Figure 1-8).

CLINICAL PEARL

A partial prism's primary action is to reduce the amplitude of the scanning eye movements into the blind field, rather than to increase awareness of the field.

A prism with the base placed in the direction of the field loss is placed over a portion of the lens in the nonseeing field. As the eye begins to scan the scotoma for an object, it passes into the prism whereupon everything is shifted toward the seeing field, lessening the size of the scanning movement to reach the object. In essence the prism allows the object to meet the eye halfway and thereby improves efficiency. Once the object is located, a head rotation returns the eye to the regular portion of the lens for an unobscured view. Because the prism is only used for locating the object and not for prolonged scrutiny, a Fresnel prism is usually acceptable to most patients for this technique. Specialty optical labs can fabricate cemented prism wafers if the patient strongly objects to the visual quality of the Fresnel.

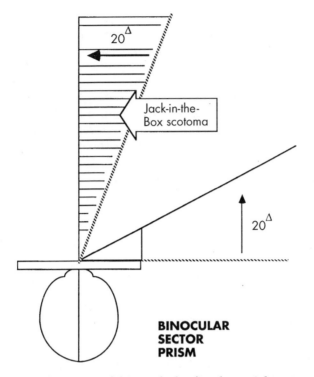

FIGURE 1-8 Schematic of binocularly fitted partial sector prisms under binocular viewing conditions. A prism jump scotoma characterizes the transition from lens to prism.

However, they are more limited in power availability relative to the Fresnel lenses and although the cementing process has improved from many years ago, the prism wafer occasionally falls off.

The two major drawbacks to the partial prism approach are the scotoma induced by the prism jump at the transition of the lens and prism edge, and the active role required of the patient for the technique to be effective. As the eye enters the prism, a scotoma is created by the shift of the optical image. The size of the scotoma will depend on the strength of the prism and the distance of the object from the prism. This results in a potential Jack-in-the-Box phenomenon which many patients find disconcerting, especially if there are cognitive deficits or slowed reaction time. The second problem is that the technique works only if the patient scans into the scotomatous fields. Patients with neglect and/or cognitive deficits may be unable to generate these scanning movements on an intentional or regular enough basis to be effective. Extensive eye scanning training is often a necessary adjunct therapy if the prism is to be useful.

The placement of the prism edge determines the size of the excursion the eye must make before it encounters the prism. The exact placement is best left to customized trial fitting procedures; however, over time two general approaches have evolved. The first is to keep the central lens clear for normal eye movement, and to place the prism in a moderately peripheral position on the lens.[7] Our philosophy, however, is to position the prism as close to the center of the lens as possible. Placement close to the center of the lens allows easier intentional access to the prism, and since occasional random eye movements enter the prism it also serves as a reminder to periodically scan the missing field even without an immediate cause for it. We have found that patients wearing the peripherally placed prism rarely use it and the perceived benefit may in reality be due to the vision training exercises that teach patients to scan into the hemianopic field to locate the prism.

Although some doctors fit the prism monocularly,[8, 9] we prefer to fit them binocularly. The monocular fit causes diplopia when the patient looks through the prism, unless the target is peripheral enough to cause the diplopic image to be occluded by the nose (Figure 1-9). The overlapping diplopic fields actually permit a larger expanse of field to be seen. However, in our experience the diplopia is confusing for most patients and there is better comfort with binocular correction.

Clinical management of partial prism. The patient sits comfortably in a chair with one eye occluded and fixates a straight ahead distance target. An index card is slowly moved from the scotomatous area toward the

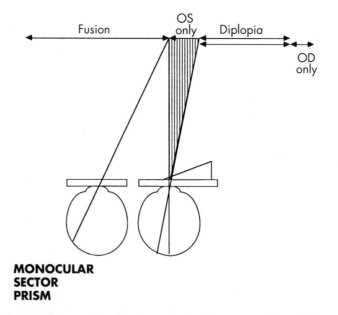

MONOCULAR
SECTOR
PRISM

FIGURE 1-9 Schematic of monocularly fit sector prism. This creates diplopia for the patient.

center of the lens until it is just seen. This position is marked on the lens. The process is repeated until a consistent finding is obtained. The occluder is switched to the other side and the sequence is duplicated on the second eye. The occluder is then removed and the positioning is checked for symmetry under binocular conditions.

A Fresnel prism with base toward the scotoma is then placed on each lens about 1 to 2 mm before the demarcation points marked on the lens. We generally start with a 15 prism diopter lens and modify the power after the most comfortable position on the lens is found. It is helpful to have precut prisms in a selection of powers for trial purposes in order to prevent the waste of unnecessarily cutting up prisms. The initial testing to determine the optimal prism placement can also be done utilizing a strip of translucent or opaque tape if necessary and gauging the patient's reactions from that.

After the prism is applied, the patient is asked to scan the environment and report on his reaction. The prism is slowly moved back off from the midline as needed until the patient is comfortable and just barely aware of the prism under these normal dynamic viewing conditions. This position is now marked and represents what we believe to be the area of the field covered by the patient's normal head and eye scanning patterns. The prism edge is set at this location.

The patient is then taught to scan into the prism to locate objects and to rotate the head to reposition the object on the clear part of the lens when necessary. Again the patient's reaction and actual performance in successfully locating objects in the room are important in deciding if this technique is suitable. The power of the prism is then varied to find the preferred strength.

The patient is then permitted to stand and try the prism while walking around. The consequences of the prism edge jump are explained and the patient is warned to be alert for them. Any final adjustment in the prism position or power should be made at this time. The Fresnel prism is then cut and applied to the lens according to the measured parameters and if all is satisfactory the patient is scheduled for appropriate follow-up.

Summary of Hemianopic Field Enhancement

The three techniques described above can help cover a wide range of patient needs and activities. Some patients respond to all three techniques and may utilize a variety of devices for various activities in their daily lives. Other patients may accept only one type of remediation, and others may find none of the techniques acceptable.

We feel that there would be more injustice to the patient if these options were never demonstrated. Clinically, all you can do is expose the patient to the device and decide if the outcome is worthwhile to pursue. Many patients are comforted by the fact that they are functioning as well as they are without these assistive devices. A device should be dispensed only if it truly helps the patient in the real world and not simply because "he has a hemianopia and this device is what is used to correct hemianopias." Also, whether the patient utilizes an optical appliance or not, it is important not to overlook the nonoptical modes of compensation. Rehabilitative vision training can help patients use their optical devices more efficiently, and teaching effective scanning techniques will help them even when no optical intervention is used.

Simple environmental modifications and ergonomic adjustments can make a world of difference in the patient's quality of life. Patient counseling and education about the visual characteristics of the condition will help the patient and the family or caretaker understand why the patient behaves the way he does. They will better understand why merely placing the silverware and tableware on the same side as the seeing field will improve the person's mealtime function. For reading, the use of line guides and margin markers, tilting the page and shifting the reading material toward the seeing field, or reinforcing the use of the patient's thumb to mark the end of each line, will likewise improve performance.

CLINICAL PEARL

Simple environmental modifications and ergonomic adjustments can make a world of difference in the patient's quality of life.

One last issue which must be addressed with regard to hemianopic patients is their driving status. We believe they should be strongly discouraged from driving despite the fact that in many states (which lack minimum field requirements) they remain legally qualified to drive. If the patient's car is outfitted with wide angle rear view and side fender mirrors (available in most auto parts stores), there are some extraordinary patients who can compensate adequately to drive safely. However, these are the rare exceptions and they still remain at high risk because of their field defect. Patients must prove their proficiency based on a thorough driving evaluation given by a neutral third party observer before approval can be reluctantly given.

Treatment of Overall Field Loss

Cases involving overall field loss are among the most frustrating because of the lack of visual material to work with. Expectations are low and results are generally limited. Every patient with constricted fields should be counseled regarding the need for a referral for an evaluation by an orientation and mobility specialist, even when the patient denies any problem with mobility.

CLINICAL PEARL

Every patient with constricted fields should be counseled regarding the need for a referral for an evaluation by an orientation and mobility specialist, even when the patient denies any problem with mobility.

Since overall field loss generally develops slowly over time, most patients develop compensatory scanning skills for extracting information from the periphery. Head swings, rapid eye sweeps of the environment, and marginally slowed approach speed allow the patient to construct the gestalt from the multiple discrete bits of input. This is all done quite naturally and the behavior is imperceptible on casual observation. The patient is usually unaware of any problem until the visual field drops to a range of about 10 degrees or less.

A perfect example is a new patient we saw recently with a history of advanced glaucoma. He came to us with a chief complaint of some recent difficulty reading and some definite but manageable orientation problems. He reported difficulty finding street signs and occasionally bumping into people. He never had orientation and mobility training and he traveled independently with no restrictions. Observation of the patient traversing the hallway and entering the exam room revealed a slightly cautious approach but there was no obvious head scanning and no major difficulty orienting to the furniture in the room. Examination revealed no light perception OD and 20/20 with a 10 degree field OS. Near complaints were solved by reducing his present +4.00 diopter add to a +3.00 diopter add. This case illustrates how well a patient can continue to function despite the loss of over 95% of the visual field.

The strategy for the treatment of overall field loss centers on increasing the amount of visual information contained in the residual island of vision and improving the efficiency and efficacy of visual scanning. The first aspect of the strategy involves minification of the image and the second involves visual training and prism.

Minification

Treating overall field loss is inversely analogous to the more familiar treatment paradigm for central field loss. In the case of central field loss, the doctor attempts to transfer information from the scotoma by magnifying it into the periphery by either decreasing the viewing distance or optically enlarging the object. In peripheral field loss the opposite occurs. The doctor attempts to transfer information from the periphery into the remaining central field via increased viewing distance and optical minification of the object.

Increased viewing distance remains the most natural and efficient means of maximizing residual field function. The patient is probably doing it in any case and it does not interfere with any compensatory scanning adaptations. However, it is limited in scope for practical reasons. It is impractical, for example, to read at 30 inches and impossible to scan a room from beyond the doorway.

The technique, however, does have application as in the case example cited. Moving the working distance from 10 to 14 inches did afford some relief for the patient's problem. Patient education is also important in this context as it prevents some well-intentioned but misinformed advisor from forcing the patient to hold the material closer so that "he can see it better".

Optical minification, in theory, is effective in providing increased field when increased working distance is not feasible (Figure 1-10), but there are several major drawbacks in practical application. First is the inverse relationship between the amount of field expansion and visual acuity. As minification increases, the visual acuity decreases in direct proportion. So although a −5X device might increase a 10 degree field to 50 degrees, the 20/20 acuity would be reduced to 20/100 through it. Even though the intent of the increased field is for short term spotting

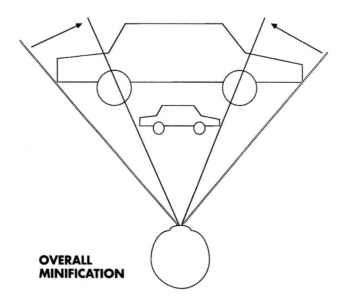

**OVERALL
MINIFICATION**

FIGURE 1-10 Schematic of overall optical minification to compact visual information to fit into the remaining reduced visual field.

purposes only (to gain a better perspective of the field), many patients will reject the device because of the poor acuity it produces.

Even more significant than the acuity loss is the disruption of the normal scanning pattern caused by the devices. Although it's true that for static viewing conditions visual field enhancers offer an increased field relative to the unenhanced eye, in the real world conditions are not static; patients scan with eye and head movements which effectively expand the range of their perceptual field to several times greater than their static visual field. Thus a patient with a 10 degree static field might have a functional field of 40 degrees while maintaining normal size constancy. Looking through a field expander cuts off the ability of the eye to freely scan space and restricts scanning movement to the field of the device itself. Often the gain in the static field through the device is offset by a loss in the dynamic functional field. Furthermore the view through the field expander is a poorly resolved, minified image compared to a normal image without the device.

Minification is achieved optically by two types of devices: reverse telescopes and minus lenses.

Reverse telescopes

Reverse telescopes utilize the same handheld monoculars and spectacle mounted telescopes used in conventional low vision protocol. There are also several low-powered minifiers, most notably by Ocutech, made specifically for field enhancement. Designs for Vision manufactures the New Horizon lens which is a series of reverse telescopes which minify in the horizontal meridian only in an attempt to preserve visual acuity.[10] Although for completeness we will show this device to patients, we have not had any positive patient response to it.

Handheld telescopes are usually worn around the neck for easy access. For patients with both decreased acuity and constricted visual fields, a handheld telescope can be used in a conventional means for standard magnification as well as reversed for orientation needs. Spectacle mounted reverse telescopes work best in bioptic form, although for stationary use, a full field position can be utilized.[11]

Clinical management of reverse telescopes. The patient sits in the exam chair and views a distant target. The patient is then given a 2.5 or 2.8X Galilean telescope and is instructed to view the scene again while looking through what is normally the objective lens of the telescope. These Galilean telescopes are lightweight, inexpensive, and easy to use while producing a bright image. Patient response is gauged regarding the overall impression of the scene viewed. If the response is positive, then other powers of telescopes are tried until the preferred telescope is chosen. The patient is coached in the concept of using the reverse telescope to scan the environment to establish the location of potential hazards and pertinent landmarks. The patient is observed for ease of use of the telescope and for improved ability to locate objects in space. The patient is also instructed that in place of eye scanning, the use of head or body rotation while maintaining focus through the telescope is the most productive way of exploring the environment through the device.

A review of the patient history and the anticipated activities for which the telescope is planned to be used should determine whether the telescope is best prescribed in handheld or spectacle mounted form. Training in use of the device is best done in conjunction with orientation and mobility personnel.

Minus Lenses

Minus lens minifiers are in principle essentially the same as reverse telescopes. The minus lens serves as the objective and patient accommodation as the ocular of a reverse telescope system. For example, if a −5.00 diopter lens is held 30 cm from the eye to view an object in the distance, the image of the minus lens would be at its focal point 20 cm in front of the lens or 50 cm from the eye (20 cm from image to lens + 30 cm from lens to eye). The patient must therefore supply 2.00 diopters in either lens form or accommodation to see this image clearly. This yields an effective telescopic power of 2/5 or 0.4 magnification which is equivalent to using the 2.5X telescope.

The advantage of the minus lens is that by tromboning the lens closer and further away, the patient changes the minification effect. The closer the minus lens is to the eye, the lower the minification; the further the minus lens is from the eye, the greater the minification.

Looking at the example of the −5.00 diopter lens, we determined that the patient obtains −2.5X when the lens is 30 cm from the eye. If it were now moved closer to 20 cm, the effective ocular would be 2.50 diopters and the magnification 2.5/5 or .5X which is equivalent to a −2X telescope. Conversely, if the lens were moved away to 47 cm, the effective ocular becomes 1.50 diopters and the magnification of the system is 1.5/5 or .3X, equivalent to a −3.3X telescope.

Minus lenses for field enhancement are available in monocle form which can be worn around the neck, but any minus lens can be used (Figure 1-11). Uncut lens blanks with a predrilled hole to thread a neck cord are an inexpensive and readily available option, as are uncut Fresnel lenses. Uncut Fresnel lenses come in a plastic frame and are lightweight and flat and fit easily into a shirt pocket. For in-office testing, trial lenses work reasonably well despite their small diameter.

For frequently viewed, large, fixed areas of space such as doorway entrances or yards and porches, large Fresnel lenses of the type used on rear van windows are extremely useful. They can be mounted on storm doors or windows overlooking the area of interest. These lenses

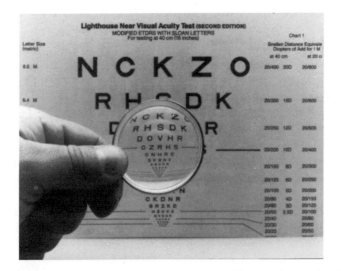

FIGURE 1-11 A minus lens creating overall optical minification.

are inexpensive and are readily available in auto supply stores and science supply houses such as Edmund Scientific.

Clinical management of minus lenses. Demonstration of minus lenses is similar to the procedure used for reverse telescopes. The patient views a distance target and then brings a minus lens up in front of the dominant sighting eye. The patient should be aware of the minified image and be instructed in tromboning the lens in and out to vary the minification. We prefer using a lens power somewhere between –5.00 to –10.00 diopters as the initial selection. This power range provides a manageable amount of minification at a reasonable lens-to-eye distance.

Once the patient is comfortable with the mechanics of using the lens, he is taught to scan the field by rotating the arm and head as a unit in order to maintain fixation through the optical axis of the lens. As the patient experiments further with the lens, different powers are introduced until a preference for power and viewing distance is demonstrated by the patient.

Enhancement of Visual Scanning Skills

While minification attempts to increase the amount of information contained in the residual field, the second approach attempts to increase the efficiency of the information gathering and input process. This can be accomplished by improved eye movement strategy and optically by prism to decrease the amplitude of the ocular excursions.

Improved eye movement strategy involves increased patient awareness of the spatial area to be processed and a plan for a systematic and complete search pattern. This type of vision therapy is best done by or in conjunction with occupational therapists and orientation and mobility instructors as its ramifications go far beyond the limits of the visual component of the patient's problems. A cooperative effort with other disciplines will decrease conflict and duplication of services and best serve the patient's interests.

Prism

As discussed earlier with hemianopic field defects, partial prisms can bring unseen visual information closer to the area of functioning field and thereby decrease the size of the scanning eye movements into the area of scotoma.

In the case of an overall field defect the residual central field is surrounded by scotoma on all sides. Therefore multiple prisms must be used to cover the different fields. How many prisms and their precise location will depend on a number of factors including the patient's binocular state, lifestyle and needs, and response to the prism.

Although occasionally a patient will manage with a single base-out prism placed temporally on each eye, covering the right and left fields respectively, two prisms placed nasally and temporally on each lens is usually the minimum number of prisms used. The maximum number is four prisms per eye, forming a ring around the central field (Figure 1-12). Remember that the prism base is always toward the scotoma, thus, the nasal prism is base-in, the temporal prism is base-out, the inferior prism is base-down, and the superior prism is base-up.

Fresnel prisms are generally used for this technique although some specialty labs will fabricate ground-in prism spectacle lenses within limited parameters. The small and often unsymmetrical visual fields of patients with overall constriction leaves room for innovative fitting approaches and leads to less uniformity in patient response as compared to other types of field loss and treatment modes. In one case report, the doctor and patient opted to split the pupil with prism touching apex to apex to achieve best results.[12]

Clinical management of prism. The patient views a distance target with the preferred eye. An index card is placed temporally on the lens and is moved in toward the lens center until it is first perceived by the patient. The process is repeated from the nasal direction and both points are marked on the lens. Two strips of 10 to 15 prism diopters of Fresnel prism are placed at those points with the bases pointing away from the lens center. The patient is then permitted to scan the room, and the position of the prism is adjusted until a comfortable central corridor is established between the prisms. The process is repeated inferiorly and, if desired, superiorly. The patient is taught to appreciate the effect of the prism and to utilize the appropriate head rotation

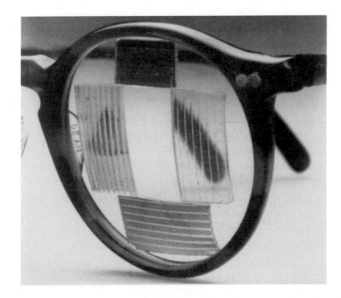

FIGURE 1-12 Circular placement of Fresnel prisms placed with the bases of the prism toward the periphery of the lens to compensate for an overall reduced visual field.

and return the eye to the home base of the clear central corridor of the lens. Changes in the strength of the prism can be made based on patient response.

The entire process is repeated on the second eye. The prisms are then checked with both eyes open with further adjustment being made on the prisms to resolve any binocular conflict. The patient is then allowed to stand and walk around with the prism. He is asked for his immediate response and again after a short trial doing a variety of distance and near centered activities. A weeklong home trial is recommended unless the patient rejects the prisms outright. At follow-up visits the prism can be refined in regard to both power and positioning.

Summary of Enhancement Techniques for Overall Visual Field Loss

Patients with overall field loss generally do not respond well to optical enhancement because of the major disruption of their normal visual equilibrium. Both techniques, minification and prisms, have limited effectiveness and considerable visual side effects. Patients coming for low vision care, however, are experiencing difficulties related to their visual deficits and will be more open to try the options offered them. It is incumbent upon the doctor to work with the patient and allow the patient the option of accepting or refusing the intervention.

As the devices described above are primarily for general orientation, special consideration must be given to reading. Obviously the patient should try to maintain the longest working distance possible to maximize the field. Weiss has suggested using a low-powered minus lens but our experience has not found great patient acceptance for it.[13] More important to patients than the small field itself is the inability to maintain one's place on the page while reading. This problem is best resolved by the use of a typoscope to keep attention focused on a small and stable but manageable area of text and to help reorient the patient should fixation be lost. When magnification is needed in order to read the paperweight-type stand magnifiers provide an exceptionally stable image and are usually well received by patients with small fields. Closed circuit televisions (CCTV) also provide a stable image for patients and offer a wide range of magnification and contrast options to the user.

Lighting and contrast enhancement are essential parameters to be discussed with patients, since the usual pathologies causing constricted fields are associated with light adaptation problems and glare sensitivity.

Conclusions

There are numerous approaches for the rehabilitation of visual field defects and each technique has both inherent flaws and advantages. The doctor should be capable of offering a selection of treatments to the patients so that they can choose the options that best fit their individual needs. The doctor must also be cognizant of the vast network of nonoptometric services available to help the patients deal with the complex difficulties associated with whatever precipitative factor has caused the field defect. It is unlikely the visual problems will be resolved unless the physical, psychological, and social needs of the patient are being met.

References

1. Cohen JM, Waiss B: An overview of enhancement techniques for peripheral field loss, J Am Optom Assoc 64(1):60-70, 1993.
2. Goodlaw E: Review of low vision management of visual field defects, Optom Mon 74(7):363-368, 1983.
3. Goodlaw E: Rehabilitating a patient with bitemporal hemianopia, Am J Optom Physio Opt 59(7):617-619, 1982.
4. Waiss B, Cohen JM: Utilization of a temporal mirror coating of the back surface of the lens as a field enhancement device, J Am Optom Assoc 63:576-580, 1992.
5. Mintz MJ: A mirror for hemianopia, Am J Ophthalmol 88:768, 1979.
6. Padula W, Shapiro JB, Jasin P: Head injury causing post trauma vision syndrome, New Eng J Opt 41(2):16-21, 1989.

7. Perlin RR, Dziadul J: Fresnel prisms for field enhancement of patients with constricted or hemianopic visual fields, *J Am Optom Assoc* 62:58-64, 1991.

8. Gottlieb DD, Freeman P, Williams M: Clinical research and statistical analysis of a visual field awareness system, *J Am Optom Assoc* 63:581-588, 1992.

9. Smith JL, Weiner IG, Lucero AJ: Hemianopic Fresnel prisms, *J Clin Neuro-ophthalmol* 2:149-158, 1982.

10. Hoeft WW, Feinbloom W, Brilliant R, et al: Amorphic lenses: A mobility aid for patients with retinitis pigmentosa, *Am J Optom Physiol Opt* 62(2):142-148, 1985.

11. Jose RT, Spitzberg LS, Kuether CL: A behind the lens reversed (BTLR) telescope, *J Vision Rehabil* 3(2):37-46, 1989.

12. Weiss NJ: An unusual application of prisms for field enhancement, *J Am Optom Assoc* 61(4):291-293, 1990.

13. Weiss NJ: Low vision management of retinitis pigmentosa, *J Am Optom Assoc* 62(1):42-52, 1991.

Appendix 1: Material Resource List*

Designs For Vision
(Amorphic Lens/Horizon Lens)
760 Koehler Avenue
Ronkonkoma, NY 11779
(800) 345-4009

Jardon Institute for Eye Care, Inc.
(clip-on hemianopic mirror)
17100 W. 12 Mile Road
Southfield, MI 48076
(313) 424-8560

Ocutech (field expanders)
P.O. Box 625
Chapel Hill, NC 27515
(919) 967-6460

Fresnel Prism and Lens Co.
(Fresnel prism)
24996 State Road 35
Siren, WI 54872
(715) 349-2638

Rekindle
(Gottlieb visual field awareness)
C/O Gottlieb Vision Group
5462 Memorial Drive, Suite 101
Stone Mountain, GA 30083
(800) 666-7484

Edmund Scientific Co.
(large minus Fresnel lenses)
101 East Gloucester Pike
Barrington, NJ 08007-1380
(609) 547-8880

Franel Optical (monocles)
P.O. Box 940096
Maitland, FL 32794
(800) 327-2070

Bernell Corp. (prism training glasses)
750 Lincolnway East
P.O. Box 4637
South Bend, IN 46634
(800) 348-2225

---

* A partial listing of available items as 11/94.

2

Eccentric Viewing

William F. O'Connell

Key Terms

eccentric viewing	scanning laser	prismatic
scotoma	ophthalmoscope	displacement
eccentric fixation	(SLO)	pleioptics
preferred retinal	perceptual filling	image remapping
locus (PRL)	pastpointing	

Eccentric viewing is an anomaly in the science of low vision care. We all have experienced patients who, on their own, have perfected the use of an eccentric fixation point in order to read around their central scotomas. For years, low vision specialists have used a variety of methods to train other patients who have *not* adapted to their central scotomas. Yet for an area of such clinical importance to the millions of individuals coping with central vision loss, there is, to risk a pun, a relative black hole when it comes to information on appropriate and efficient training techniques for eccentric viewing. The clinical importance of current and past research is highlighted when we consider that ARMD accounts for roughly 13% of patients registered as legally blind.[1]

The purpose of this chapter is twofold: to bring practitioners up to date on past research into eccentric viewing training and to provide practical training techniques that can be used now, in the office, based upon new research done. This chapter will also suggest areas where further research needs to be done.

What Is Eccentric Viewing?

The fovea has a diameter of approximately 5 degrees, with the central 1.2 to 1.7 degrees known as the foveola or rod free area.[2] In the healthy retina the center of this zone is the area used for fixation. When the central retina is damaged the eye must choose a new retinal area to view with.

The terms *eccentric viewing* and *eccentric fixation* have been used somewhat interchangeably to describe the use of any nonfoveal point on the retina for viewing, yet they have slightly different meanings. In eccentric fixation, patients have the sensation of looking directly at the fixation target, whereas in eccentric viewing, patients realize that they are looking away in order to see the fixation target.[2] Some patients who use eccentric viewing may use a nonfoveal point to aim the eye, and others may use the fovea by intentionally aiming it off to one side to allow functioning retina to see the target.[3]

CLINICAL PEARL

In eccentric fixation, patients have the sensation of looking directly at the fixation target.

CLINICAL PEARL

In eccentric viewing, patients realize that they are looking away in order to see the fixation target.

Eccentric viewing and eccentric fixation occur in many strabismus and amblyopia cases. There, it is an undesirable phenomenon which we attempt to correct with vision training to reorient fixation onto the center of the macula or fovea. Although this is the opposite of what we try to do with patients who have macular degeneration, many of the training techniques developed for amblyopia and strabismus cases may be used to help patients deal with macular scotomas.

What Is a Scotoma?

A scotoma is a "blind spot" resulting from injury, disease, or degeneration of retinal photoreceptors, the optic pathway, or the visual cortex. In reality, what we refer to as a scotoma may be vastly different presenting symptoms to our patients. The area not functioning properly may have some residual function with simply a loss of detail. It may be seen as a fogged area with whitish, grayish, black, or even colored appearance, or it may be truly a blind or black spot in the visual field.

Frequently patients are unaware that scotomas exist. They may complain that small objects vanish and jump back into view, that parts of objects, signs, and words are missing or blurry, but they do not realize that the reason for these phenomena is a scotoma.[2] Scotomas may be relative or absolute.

Research has shown that scotomas are associated with 64% of reading speed variations.[4] The scotomas at or near the center of patients' visual fixation are those we strive to deal with clinically when we train eccentric viewing.

Why Do Some Patients Eccentrically View on Their Own While Others Do Not?

Many patients with macular retinal lesions adapt on their own over varying periods of time, and learn to use areas in the retinal periphery to view their environment. Although younger patients with hereditary or congenital conditions are far more likely to adapt successfully than are older patients with years of having used the macula for fixation, many older patients appear to adapt quite readily. The fact that younger patients adapt well is seemingly easy to accept, but the success of some older patients (even into their eighth decade of life), while other patients are unsuccessful even after extensive attempts at training, is less easy to explain.

When the central retina is damaged, the eye must choose a new retinal area for viewing. Many researchers feel that this new point is arrived at naturally with no intervention needed.[2] Research on monkeys who had bilateral foveal lesions artificially induced by laser showed that they developed a new preferred retinal locus (PRL) within days, although it was weeks to months before they were able to develop their eye movements to accurately place targets in their PRL.[2]

CLINICAL PEARL

When the central retina is damaged, the eye must choose a new retinal area for viewing.

Clinically, however, many patients (particularly older patients) have apparently not found a PRL and need to be taught that they have a scotoma and can view around it. These patients may already view eccentrically, but may be embarrassed to do so until you demonstrate it and explain that it is not only acceptable but the preferred thing to do.[5] If you were to ask each patient, after demonstrating eccentric viewing, if they had ever done this on their own, some believe the answer would nearly always be yes.[5]

Examination

Assessment of Patients

A careful assessment is necessary to determine the needs and problems of a given patient. A careful assessment begins in the waiting room when the patient is greeted. Does the patient look you in the eyes, look off to the side in a consistent direction, or simply stare blankly out into space? How did the patient behave while waiting? Did the patient look actively around the room to become oriented, simply sit and perform no visual investigation at all, or read a book while waiting? Observation of the patient continues throughout the introduction and travel to the examination room.

While the patient's ability and desire to read is a fundamental issue, the problem is that, at this point, it is difficult to differentiate the patient's problems into those that can be solved simply with appropriate magnification versus those requiring an eccentric viewing application.

Some indications can be found by in-depth questioning that may reveal more difficulty with continuous text reading as compared to single letters and words. Patients may also report that they frequently have difficulty reading large print and headlines because certain letters are regularly missing. In addition, difficulty seeing faces and signs may indicate central lockup difficulties. Patients with central vision loss of moderate degree who also complain of mobility problems (rare in this class of patients) may be signaling the need for eccentric viewing training.

Visual acuity

The first clinical test performed can often provide valuable information about the patient's status. Clinical presentation is variable, but typically patients locking on their scotoma will read nothing on their own, necessitating the clinician to begin chart-jumping or suddenly moving the acuity chart up-down or right-left in order for the patient to see the figure. This level of impairment generally occurs only with acuities significantly below 20/200 and more often below 20/400, although an occasional patient with better acuity may present this way. Usually with better than 20/400 acuities, the patient will consistently miss one or more letters on the chart, often following a pattern such as missing numbers to the right, the left, or in the center.

It is important that with the first group, single figures be used to test acuity on a handheld chart to allow rapid chart movement. The Designs for Vision or a similar chart is best suited for this purpose. When moving the chart elicits the desired response, try moving the chart in different directions to see which directions work best. Then shift strategies and instead of moving the chart, have the patient look away in the opposite direction indicated by the chart-jumping, preferably without moving the head, until the figure comes into view.

With the second group, an EDTRS type chart such as the Lighthouse acuity chart (Figure 2-1) is preferred because of the consistency in figure spacing as the letters or numbers get smaller.

Clinically, it is best to take time during testing to discuss the way the patient reads the chart if either of the above two types of reading are apparent. This is the first opportunity to discuss the nature of the patient's condition and what you will be attempting to do about it.

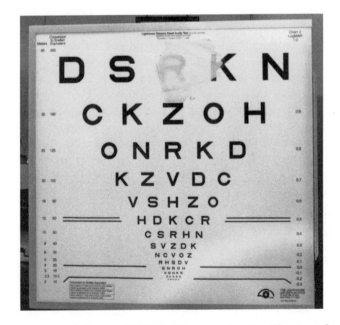

FIGURE 2-1 Lighthouse ETDRS Distance Acuity Chart with simulated scotoma.

Scotoma awareness

During acuity testing, it is helpful to ascertain the patient's awareness of the scotoma, and whether or not any tendency is shown to control the scotoma and eccentrically view.

Patients clinically range from individuals who lock up on a scotoma badly yet have no idea that there is a scotoma present, to those who very successfully use eccentric viewing and yet have no idea how or why, and also do not visualize the scotoma. It is important to question patients about their perceptions as this can be a logical starting point for training. Education is in order for both of these types of patients. On the other end of the spectrum, awareness of the scotoma does not ensure success.

Amsler grid

Although it is often considered a valuable predictive test for scotoma-related problems, this test also has significant shortcomings. Patients with large visible scars in the macular area will report a normal Amsler grid nearly as often as they will identify the scotoma. They appear to perceptually fill in the image on some cortical level even though we as clinicians realize that what they report cannot be so.[6]

Schuchard (1993) tested patients on the scanning laser ophthalmoscope (SLO) and found that the sensitivity of both standard and threshold Amsler grid testing was very low, failing to detect almost half of all scotomas. Even when the scotomas are detected on the Amsler grid test, the full extent of the scotoma is frequently understated.[6] In addition, more than 65% of patients placed their preferred retinal locus at the center of the grid, giving the false illusion of a paracentral scotoma rather than one affecting the fovea.[7] Unless the exact location of the PRL is known, it is impossible to use the information to judge the size and shape of the scotoma.[6] The study found that the larger a scotoma was, the more likely it was to be detected.[6]

CLINICAL PEARL

The sensitivity of both standard and threshold Amsler grid testing was very low, failing to detect almost half of all scotomas.

Several means exist to try to elicit more accurate responses to this test. First, some patients will visualize the scotoma better if they are allowed to see the relative changes that occur from a binocular presentation to a monocular one. Even in patients with similar acuities and scotomas, they can often see the difference when one eye is occluded. For this reason, some clinicians will test the Amsler grid binocularly first and then occlude each eye in turn. Second, using thresh-old illumination techniques, either by using a light dimmer, rotating Polaroid lenses, or Amsler grids of different colors (particularly red or of lower contrast), may assist the patient in visualizing the scotoma.

Given these potential problems and realizing their import, the ability or inability to view the scotoma gives little insight into the training needed for a particular patient. Additionally, the location of the scotoma when it is visualized gives little information about the patient's ability to eccentrically view. Little information is produced as to whether patients realize they are eccentrically viewing or not, the direction of eccentric viewing, or the position of the scotoma. Scoto-mas that appear to the right of fixation are logically going to be more problematic since most European languages, including English, in-volve reading from left to right.

This pattern of perceptual filling in of the grid by most patients indicates the need for a new test for macular function.[1] In the meanwhile, we cannot count heavily on the accuracy of results of this common test.

Contrast sensitivity

Contrast sensitivity testing, while covered more thoroughly in other chapters, can also have its clinical implications in determining the need for eccentric viewing training and its potential outcome. When central scotomas exist there is a significant difference in testing with VCTS type targets which contain small circles that may be smaller than the scotoma, versus testing with TV type tests where the field of the grid is large enough compared to the scotoma size to allow measurement of contrast sensitivity in the surrounding retina. The binocular versus monocular findings may also indicate whether or not occlusion is indicated.

Research done by Rubin found that while contrast is important for many other everyday activities, in the case of reading, for normal subjects with letters of near optimal size, contrast drops of tenfold reduced reading speed by a factor of less than two.[1] For visually impaired readers, the effect of contrast is far greater, with many fast readers unable to read at all if contrast fell below 30%.[1]

CLINICAL PEARL

For visually impaired readers, the effect of contrast is far greater, with many fast readers unable to read at all if contrast fell below 30%.

Contrast polarity was found to be a factor particularly for patients with cloudy media where reverse contrast was found to be of benefit.

Other causes of low vision found patients varying widely in their responses, although when there was a preference it was almost always for reverse contrast. Normally sighted readers tend to read about 10% faster with conventional black on white lettering.[1]

Binocularity and dominance

Clinically we see many patients with a strong dominance in the eye with poorer acuity or the larger scotoma. There are also cases where the acuity may be nearly equal, but the shape of the scotoma or the eccentric viewing position for a particular favored eye is less favorable for reading continuous text than the position in the other eye. It is important that both eyes are tested monocularly and binocularly when possible, on actual continuous text tasks.

Often the patient's performance may be better binocularly than it is with either eye monocularly. When this occurs every attempt should be made to facilitate binocular viewing, although the only methods to allow this with higher magnifications are currently the CCTV and Low Vision Enhancement System (LVES).

Single symbol vs. single word vs. continuous text acuities

If the patient's principal goal is to read, the near acuity testing is often the most definitive indicator of potential scotoma-related difficulties. The way we test patients' acuity, however, will determine just how useful the information will be.

There are valid reasons to test with single figures, single words, and continuous text; and your clinical regimen may justifiably include all three. If the patient's goal includes reading, however, you have not done a full exam without testing for continuous text acuity. There are many charts available for this, with the Lighthouse continuous text acuity cards presently being the most popular. The key things to look for are varying print sizes down to those sizes smaller than the size of the print the patient desires to read. Short passages at a grade level the patient can easily read are best. The Lighthouse continuous text reading cards are ideal for measurement of continuous text acuity. Because the text passages are shorter and clearly at a grade level that is obtainable by most readers, it is often best to use the children's version of the card (Figure 2-2).

CLINICAL PEARL

If the patient's goal includes reading, however, you have not done a full exam without testing for continuous text acuity.

Lastly, the optimum test for all patients is to have them read the types of materials they desire to read on a daily basis. There are

LIGHTHOUSE "CONTINUOUS TEXT" CARD FOR CHILDREN
FOR NEAR VISION
LINE INCREMENTS IN LIGHTHOUSE FONTS

| | SNELLEN EQUIV ALENT | 1/8 YRK PHPUT SV/I |

The hen was sitting on the shed.   20/160   3.2M

Patty spilled some jam on the rug.   20/125   2.5M

I will make a wish for a red pen.   20/100   2.0M

The big circus cats ran in the cage.   20/80   1.6M

A pet shop is a nice place to visit.   20/60   1.25M

The children took Grandma some flowers.   20/50   1.0M

My dog likes to play catch with a stick   20/40   8M

The sense of fun I know the funny things   20/30   6M

I see lots a bird that says the size his bell fly around the track 20/25   5M

h m r i i m in arm a tr me can art   20/20   4M

THIS CARD IS CALIBRATED FOR USE AT 40 CM OR IN WITH CUSTOMARY READING CORRECTION IF NEEDED
LIGHTHOUSE™ LOW VISION PRODUCTS 36-02 NORTHERN BLVD LONG ISLAND CITY, N.Y. 11101   ©1989
CAT. NO. C 212

FIGURE 2-2 Lighthouse "continuous text" card for children.

considerable differences between high quality charts and poor quality
print such as that found in newspapers.

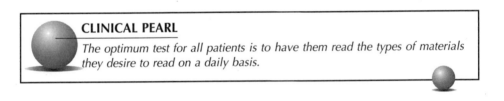

CLINICAL PEARL

*The optimum test for all patients is to have them read the types of materials
they desire to read on a daily basis.*

Pastpointing

Eccentric fixation may produce pastpointing, where a patient monocularly may point to one side or the other of a penlight held at 40 cm by
the doctor. Patients can be trained to compensate for this easily and
often have learned on their own. In order to test for pastpointing and
avoid the compensating movements for eye-hand coordination, use an
opaque card with vertical lines drawn in the same location on both
sides. Have the patient use a pointer to touch the position of the line
on the back side of the card. The angle of pastpointing can be easily
calculated by measurement.[8] One measurement technique involves
using an Amsler grid with a hole cut in it to shine a light through.

Acuity predictions

The patient's best acuity with eccentric viewing also provides some
information about the angle from the fovea to the eccentric viewing
point. This is illustrated in several charts.[2,8] The chart in Wetter et al

depicts the acuity relative to disc diameters from the fovea for normal and macular diseased eyes,[2] while Griffen uses degrees of eccentricity for normal and amblyopic eyes.[8] They are only of value if the exact position and size of the scotoma is known (as in scanning laser ophthalmoscopy) and if the exact viewing point is known, since later research pointed out that the selected viewing point was not always the one closest to the fovea. For that reason, the charts are not reprinted here.

Visuoscopy

This technique involves the use of a direct ophthalmoscope with a fixation target for the patient. When the target is fixated by a nonfoveal point outside the macula it is possible to note the direction of this position, the steadiness of fixation, and (if the calibration of the rings surrounding the target is known) an approximate angle of eccentricity.[8]

Fundus photography

While the techniques may not be readily available or practical for all clinical situations, the fundus camera shows promise as a research tool and as a way of documenting the eccentric viewing position of a particular patient. The patient is instructed to look directly at a fixation target in the fundus camera. The photograph that results then shows the area on the retina that corresponds to the fixation target as well as the size and shape of the damaged retinal area.

   If video viewing were possible, much more information would be available and the needed retinal illumination could be provided in a manner that would allow comfort for the patient. Video fundus cameras using infrared illumination are one possible solution.

Scanning laser ophthalmoscopy (SLO)

The most promising new technology currently available involves the scanning laser ophthalmoscope with graphics capabilities. In this instrument, the retina is scanned with an infrared (780 nm) laser over an area of either 32×22 degrees or 16×11 degrees. The image provided is extremely sharp and the infrared source causes no discomfort to the patient. Graphics of virtually unlimited variety may be placed on the retina at any position within the fields viewed using a low-power visible red (633 nm) laser. The strength of the stimulus is variable in 256 steps from 50 to 50,000 trolands. This setup allows the user to view the retina while testing the fields to accurately measure the edges of the scotoma. In addition, the patient can be tested while actually viewing a variety of presented targets in order to determine the location of the eccentric viewing point (also known as the preferred retinal locus or PRL). The patient's PRL can then be monitored while reading presented text to see if the PRL is adequate to the task or if the type and position of the nearby scotoma(s) prevent reading with the existing PRL and perhaps indicate another nearby spot that may perform better.

While this is the "hottest technology on the block" at present, there are many reasons to hold off at least for now. First, the studies so far do not clearly indicate that this accurate measurement is essential to help train eccentric viewing. Many low vision specialists are able to help the majority of their patients with no blind spot measurement being done at all. The technology will clearly help us with the more difficult cases in the future, by pointing to a PRL point that may be superior. However, that does not necessarily mean that the patient will succeed, as there are many other factors that enter into patient success. The cost of the instrument, the expertise required to use it, and the time required to do the testing are prohibitive for practical use in every low vision service at this time. Our patients often cannot afford a needed magnifier and the fees we can charge these patients are in many cases already too low to provide the level of services we would like to provide to every patient. A better recommendation is to have the instrument available in regional referral centers so that motivated patients who do not respond well to conventional techniques may be sent for thorough evaluation. Expensive instrumentation that is time-consuming to use is not going to be the answer for most patients, at least in the near future.

Tangent screen/autoplot/other field tests

Visual field tests used to measure the size, shape, and position of the patient's scotoma can be valuable in plieoptic training, research, and planning for an eccentric viewing locus. Careful measurement calls for the largest available screen, preferably a one- or two-meter tangent screen and/or autoplot. An "X" may be used to aid in fixation control.

Goodrich and Quillman believed that the low vision specialist should know the patient's precise visual field as measured on a tangent screen, and the patient's visual acuity. In general they believed in training the intact visual field to the center of the fovea, since this area should have the best visual acuity and the sharpest image.[9]

The shortcoming of any visual field test is that it is impossible to know the actual position of the patient's preferred retinal locus. In addition the size and shape of the measured scotoma may vary as much as 5 degrees due to fluctuations in the PRL position and in the blind spot, if this is being used as a fixation check. These variations may result in errors of greater than 5 degrees.[6]

Studies using the SLO have indicated that actual scotomas range from 3 to 30 degrees larger than measured on a tangent screen with even well-adapted patients, although scotoma shapes tended to agree well.[6] In other words, all field tests are limited at best in giving field information reliable enough to base eccentric viewing training on.

> **CLINICAL PEARL**
>
> *Actual scotomas range from 3 to 30 degrees larger than measured on a tangent screen with even well-adapted patients, although scotoma shapes tended to agree well.*

Patient Selection—Motivation

A critical but often overlooked area in examining and planning treatment/therapy is motivation. The process of learning how to read again with an eccentric retinal area is time-consuming and frustrating. The average patient may not have the necessary desire and motivation to go through this process. It is important to assess not only the patient's goals in a thorough history, but also to assess just how badly the patient wants to reach these goals (a much more difficult task). In addition the clinician periodically needs to reassess the patient's motivation to continue, and should actively work to keep the patient's motivation levels high through encouragement and reasonable goal setting.

> **CLINICAL PEARL**
>
> *The process of learning how to read again with an eccentric retinal area is time-consuming and frustrating.*

Awareness and Ability to Follow Complex Instructions and Understand the Concepts Involved

In addition to motivation, the patient needs to grasp the often abstract concepts involved in eccentric viewing, consistently follow the instructions, and retain the memory to take the information home and use it in day-to-day reading. Stroke, illness, simple forgetfulness, and certainly any organic degenerative cortical processes may work against success with these patients. On the other hand, persistence and motivation have yielded success with some patients who by all indications had little chance of success.

While it is theoretically possible to train eccentric viewing with a patient who does not fully understand it, a thorough understanding of the concepts and science involved is probably a significant advantage.

Training Eccentric Viewing

There are many approaches that have been used to train patients with eccentric viewing. All techniques have the potential for success when used with the appropriate patient and properly administered. A discussion of all techniques reported in the literature will be presented here.

Prismatic Displacement

A 1983 study by Romayananda et al appeared to show nearly miraculous vision improvements in almost all macular degeneration patients tested. This success was achieved with far less magnification than would be expected by any experienced clinician. Unfortunately, this work was greatly flawed in its lack of basic knowledge of low vision and weak in its application of basic optical and magnification principles. It is still known as one of the classic case reports on prismatic displacement. The work presented was never duplicated in any center nationally, but it did spark considerable interest and study of the techniques presented.

The following technique was used. They began with a reading distance of 20 cm and a 6 diopter sphere applied over the spherical equivalent of the better eye (regardless of acuity, or the fact that 20 cm is the reciprocal of 5 diopters). Then a 4 diopter prism was inserted in front while the other eye was occluded. The axis was rotated by the examiner or the patient to the position at which the reading material was clear. If clarity was not achieved, stronger prisms of 5 to 10 diopters were tried until the best visual response was received. (Most patients were noted to do best with 6 or 8 prism diopters.) The prescription was determined by successive addition of plus or minus in half diopter steps until the patient saw the print size clearly.[10]

The work of Romayananda et al was subsequently criticized by some investigators. Part of the problem in prior research has been that patients, their psychological makeup, visual acuity, size regularity, and borders of their scotomas all vary extensively.

Rosenberg, Faye, Fischer, and Budick, checking Romayananda's study, using 8 prism diopters as the first prism power choice. Some evidence was found to support prism relocation although the results were not as dramatic as the original study.[11] Bailey, in reviewing the study, found that "There is no reason to believe that the eye will change its habitual centric or eccentric viewing behavior just because. . .the prism is used."[12]

As mentioned previously, the work of Romayananda et al appears to be greatly flawed in that the results have not been repeated, even by some of the more avid supporters of the technique. That does not mean that the research was totally wasted, however, since it stimulated much interest in this underresearched area, and the techniques, while perhaps not frequently yielding prescribable results, may have some value in training patients how to eccentrically view.

Most investigators working with the prisms have found that the effect lasts for shorter than a few hours duration. Prism image relocation can be and has been shown to be effective in training eccentric viewing. Showing patients that they can see better than they thought is a useful way to introduce more difficult patients to the premise of eccentric viewing. It may also assist patients in selecting an appropriate off center spot with which to fixate. Many practitioners will use this as a backup technique when conventional training techniques have not been useful. Another reason it is not used more as a primary training technique is that it is time-consuming and generally requires the doctor to do the testing and training personally.

Training Techniques for Distance Eccentric Viewing

In addition to the prismatic relocation technique just described, there are other techniques that have been successful in helping to train patients. A list of techniques, while not exhaustive, follows below. It is important when selecting techniques to remain flexible and consider the patient in any program. Many techniques can be performed at home by some patients, especially with adequate support from family and friends. Other patients will require in-office training either because they do not readily grasp the concepts, or they have no support at home.

Blind spot awareness

Before patients can learn to eccentrically view, or look around the blind spot, they must simply be aware that they have one. For many patients this awareness is strong before they come to the office. For others, however, the blind spot is unfamiliar; they simply know that they cannot see well. It is helpful in training when the patient is aware of and able to visualize the scotoma.[13]

Some of the methods that have been considered helpful are:
1. Amsler grid (with rotating double Polaroids or colored grids if needed). If perceptual fill-in occurs other techniques must be used.
2. Observation. If patients consistently miss numbers or letters in a certain area on the chart, remind them that this is the blind spot.
3. Face observation. Sometimes the human face is helpful because details of the face are missing. It also provides a target of very low contrast. Jose outlines a typical technique for training using the face for both awareness and control training. First patch one eye, then the instructor's face is properly illuminated about two to three feet away. The patient is instructed to look directly at the face and told that "When you look at my face, some portion of it will appear unclear or missing. Can you tell me which area?" An advantage is that the instructor can clearly observe eccentric fixation if present at this close distance. Control and direction of eccentric viewing can also be trained using the face when indicated.[14]

Blind spot control

Once a patient is aware of the existence of the scotoma, it is important to begin to reinforce the use of and position of this area by having the patient purposefully use it to make things disappear. The conscious control of the scotoma will be strengthened, even though at this point the visual improvement desired as an end point will not be evident. Freeman and Jose discuss using a patch with a small 2 cm hole, where eccentric viewing becomes an "all or nothing" phenomenon. If the scotoma looks through the hole, nothing is seen whereas, eccentric viewing will yield an image. "This procedure reinforces the ocular muscles to develop a sense of directionalization to visual stimuli and in time and with effort, students develop localization skills."[15] This was discussed as being a particularly helpful technique for patients who need help looking through telescopes.

Eccentric viewing direction and degree

Once the patient can readily control and position the scotoma, it is practical to begin training designed to locate the best possible retinal tissue remaining. Although there are many variations, the general technique is to have the patient sit at a comfortable distance from an uncluttered wall with a single suprathreshold size number taped on it. (Photocopies of large numbers from various charts work well.) The patient is instructed to first look slowly to the right and then to the left, noting if he or she can see the figure in each direction, comparing which direction gave the clearer image and how far it was necessary to look in each direction. Then the patient proceeds, two at a time with eight cardinal directions comparing a new direction to the previous best of the viewing directions tested. Once the best direction and distance are found, the patient is to record the results and begin to use them consistently in practice.

Some clinicians believe that vertical viewing points should be used routinely unless there is a dramatic difference between horizontal and vertical results.[16] This is based on the practical safety problems encountered when patients cross streets. Moving the blind spot in the horizontal plane may allow the patient to see one car and think it is safe to cross after that car passes. Meanwhile another car may have fallen into the scotoma while viewing the first car, presenting a danger to the patient.

Goodrich et al. found that the consistent use of one retinal locus is easier for patients to learn, but there are no data to indicate whether this approach is the most beneficial to the patient.[17] Many patients will present with a PRL already selected, and some may have more than one PRL. Many researchers believe that it is not possible in most cases to easily retrain the patient to use another PRL. Keep this in mind when testing for the best position.

Eye-Hand Coordination—Its Relation to Eccentric Viewing

Many patients during early adaptation of a new PRL will develop eye-hand coordination problems. These are manifested by patients reporting they are spilling things and having problems picking up small objects. It is important, both for helping the patient to overcome these difficulties and to aid the patient in successfully developing eccentric viewing for reading and other activities, that this problem is met with appropriate rehabilitative efforts. Freeman recommends training using hand-over-hand activities based on trying to redevelop appropriate perspective from the new PRL to the midline of the body and to develop eye-hand coordination for the new retinal locus. When the patient grabs for something, put the object on the patient's midline; the patient will turn the head and/or eyes to the functional midline and may grab in that direction. The patient may also overcompensate in another direction. You can demonstrate this for yourself with prisms. To get the patient to acclimate to the object add multiple activities including pouring, filling in circles, pegboard rotator (Figure 2-3, D), Michigan tracking series, Marsden ball, (Figure 2-3, E) and any number of other standardized training techniques borrowed from vision training. These eye-hand recoordination training activities help define the eccentric viewing point in relation to the patient's body.

Saccadic and Pursuit Movements with Eccentric Viewing

Most training programs incorporate some exercises where the patient practices both saccadic and following eye movements with the eccentric viewing point. Any training program such as this is designed to reinforce the eccentric viewing point and to acclimate the patient to its use. The eventual goal is to try to make eccentric viewing a nearly automatic "reflex".

Researchers who believe that the selection of a PRL is a natural reaction to scotoma development believe that the real training that is done with these patients is not to aid them in finding the PRL but rather to help them develop the motor skills needed to read with this new point.

Freeman and Jose have produced a text with many preset training exercises that are useful to begin with.[15] Some of these can be duplicated on a computer using various sizes of text and can be customized to many uses, including foreign language versions.

Cummings et al. proposed measuring baseline visual skills, and using them to measure progress. They recommended that three skills be measured: (1) fixation, the ability to maintain the PRL between saccades, (2) localization, the ability to find the beginning point in text, and (3) scanning, the ability to read without skipping words or losing place.[18] They found a relationship between increasing scotoma size and reduced reading speed.

Rubin's studies of eye movements with normal viewers found the eyes making saccadic movements with pauses of about .25 seconds between saccades.[19] This resulted in a reading rate of about 240 words per minute if regressive eye movements and skipping of shorter words were ignored. By presenting words sequentially at the same location in the visual field, normal readers were able to read in excess of 1000 words per minute, suggesting that conventional reading speeds are limited by eye movement delays. In patients with scotomas, reading is generally limited to 25 to 50 words per minute. The saccades may play some role because these patients make much smaller saccades, undershooting the intended targets, and also make many more regressive saccades. A study using normally sighted individuals with text positioned by an optical stabilizer at 10 degrees eccentricity found that reading speed dropped to about 50 words per minute, similar to patients with central scotomas. Because the text images were stabilized, eye movements could not be a factor, suggesting that "peripheral vision is inherently slower at processing complex visual information like text." This research suggests that the eye movements are not an issue and that training to improve the eye movements of patients with a scotoma may have limited potential for success, and perhaps be of no benefit at all.

Whittaker et al. measured three other aspects of fixational stability and found that with scotomas of less than 20 degrees, fixation eye movements were not likely to interfere with reading.[20]

Clearly, the jury is out on this aspect of training. Clinicians are getting promising results even though preliminary research seems to indicate that they should not.

CLINICAL PEARL

Clinicians are getting promising results even though preliminary research seems to indicate that they should not.

Pleioptics

Holcomb and Goodrich used pleioptic training in their training program. The technique used has the patient seated in front of a tangent screen with a fixation aid. A threshold letter is moved about to find the point of sharpest vision and the desired viewing angle is determined by triangulation. The threshold letter is recalibrated for a 50 cm distance and is affixed to the center of a vertical strobe. The strobe is then held at the approximate angle of eccentricity indicated by the tangent screen testing and flashed, placing a negative afterimage of the letter at the patient's best visual point monocularly. The patient practices placing this afterimage on various targets at a 1 meter distance.[9] The goals are to increase speed of locating the desired target and increase time of steady fixation. As the speed and steadiness increase, task difficulty increases by having the subject follow moving targets with the afterimage. Variations of increasing difficulty are added to maintain patient interest.[21]

Training Techniques

Guided Practice Techniques

Saccade training

A distance saccade training technique uses threshold letters separated by 6 feet. They may be adjusted for vertical, horizontal, and oblique angles. It is used at 5 to 10 feet with a threshold size target at the ends of the bar. The patient looks back and forth, eccentrically fixating on each one and finally tracks the targets with a finger as they are viewed. An alternative to this is to use Design For Vision's driver training strips of letters and numbers (Figure 2-3, A).

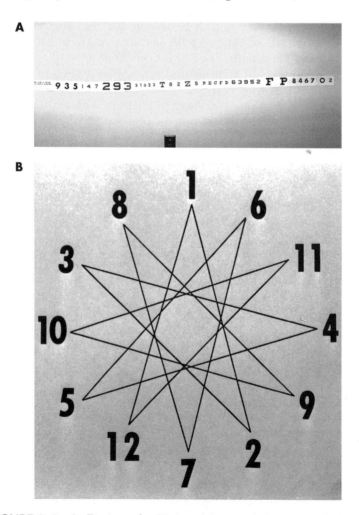

FIGURE 2-3 **A,** Designs for Vision driver training strip. **B,** Numbers arranged in a clock setup for eccentric viewing training.

Clock directions

Construct a large clock face 2 to 3 feet diameter, attach threshold figures to the outside perimeter of the clock and have the patient view them at random by calling out clock positions and having the patient identify the number at that clock position.[9] You can modify the clock by placing it on a rotator with numbers for tracking exercises. Most clinicians actually use eight directions rather than twelve (Figure 2-3, *B*).

Rotator (Keystone View Co.)

The rotator is helpful in teaching visual tracking, fixation, and pursuit to the low vision patient. The target is a small red light affixed to the edge of a rotating disc.[9] The patient follows the light with a finger, consistently using the best retinal area. The rotator may be used in both clockwise and counterclockwise directions (Figure 2-3, *C*).

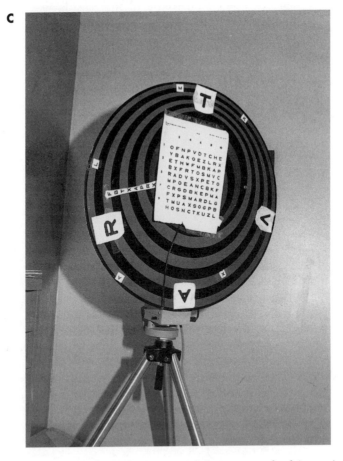

FIGURE 2-3, cont'd. C, Rotator with letters attached in periphery.
Continued

Pegboard rotator

The standard pegboard rotator used in vision training of children, is also useful for eccentric viewing training. Various targets can be placed on the rotator to elicit pursuit movement training, and placement of pegs into holes can aid in correction of pastpointing problems and remediation of eye-hand coordination difficulties (Figure 2-3, *D*).

Slide projector

Targets of differing sizes and familiarity can be flashed onto a screen for the patient to identify.[9] This training is designed to exercise the ability of the peripheral retina to identify targets.

In addition many devices utilized heavily in vision training and sports vision may be utilized. Two examples of this are the Marsden Ball (Figure 2-3, *E*) and the Wayne Saccadic Fixator (Figure 2-3, *F*). Targets swinging or flashing in the periphery, requiring the eye to fixate them and the hand to hit them, train pursuit and saccadic eye movements and eye-hand coordination. This can be further modified by placing letters, numbers, and words on or near some of the targets.

Reading—Is It the Best Training Technique?

There is no question that the best overall training for reading is the act of reading itself. When reading of small print is not possible, appro-

D

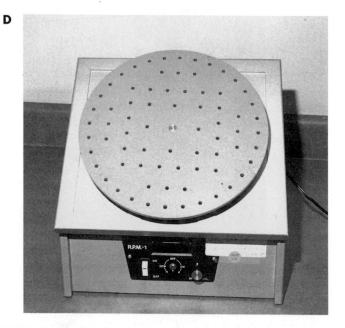

FIGURE 2-3, cont'd.   D, Pegboard for eye-hand coordination training at near.

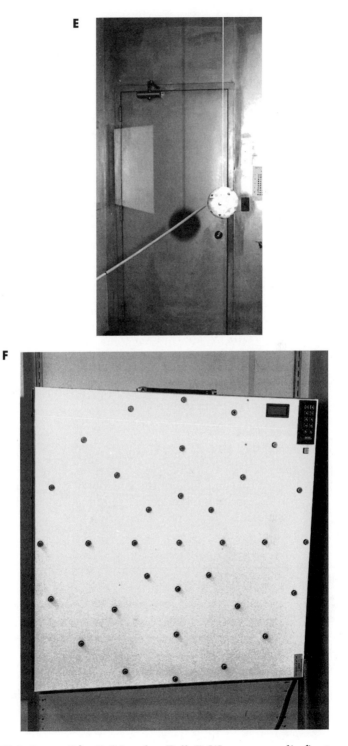

FIGURE 2-3, cont'd. E, Marsden Ball. F, Wayne saccadic fixator.

priate magnification may assist the patient in beginning the task of reading. The level of magnification may require in some cases the use of large print or the use of devices such as the CCTV.

Direction of eccentricity

Peli's work appears to confirm clinical experience that there are fewer training problems when the locus used is not along the axis of image motion.[22] This means vertical eccentric viewing is preferable unless the patient is to read Chinese.

The English alphabet

Preliminary research by Goodrich appears to indicate that patients can derive more information from the upper half of letters than from the lower half.[23] This would seem to support moving the blind spot down to allow for better reading if the scotoma was not to be entirely clear of the letters.

CCTV

For those patients with severe vision loss and for those patients experiencing poor results from initial attempts at eccentric viewing training, the CCTV can give some positive feedback and reassurance that reading is still possible. The high levels of magnification available from the CCTV allow reading for all but the most severely impaired patients. It has been used as an early eccentric viewing training tool in some of the more difficult cases.

Large print

One of the keys to long term success is to give the patient achievable goals that will cause less frustration. Large print is a useful tool toward this end. One of the benefits of computers is that they enable you to print training materials in numerous point sizes and fonts with repeatable accuracy on a laser printer.

CLINICAL PEARL

One of the keys to long term success is to give the patient achievable goals that will cause less frustration.

Commercially available large print is available from the *New York Times* (weekly), the *Readers Digest* (monthly and condensed books), the *World at Large* (bimonthly news magazine), and Christian publications.

Specialized training sheets

A good basic selection of training sheets is available in *The Art and Practice of Low Vision* by Freeman and Jose.[15] The exercises include training in selection of a vertical eccentric viewing point, tracking, and random letter and word reading exercises. Sheets with lines above and below letters, words, and continuous text are readily available in Freeman and Jose's text,[15] or they may be produced easily on the computer (Figure 2-4). The lines are designed as a reference to aid the patient in moving the scotoma above or below the line of print.[17]
SINGLE LETTERS/NUMBERS—For a simple starting point.
SMALL WORDS—Beginning with two and three letters progressing through four, five, and six letter words.
NONSENSE—RANDOM WORDS—Make the task less predictable and more difficult as the patient may not infer the correct word out of context.[8] Again, the computer with a laser printer is perfect for producing a huge variety of high quality training tools in virtually limitless point sizes (Figure 2-5).

Use of fingers/fixation aids

For patients having difficulty with pastpointing, localization, and saccades, using a reading guide such as a ruler, typoscope, or the

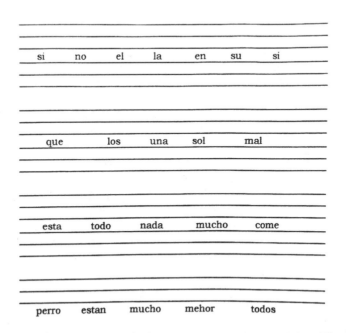

FIGURE 2-4 Random words for eccentric viewing training. The lines above and below are designed to allow the patient to find and maintain the best vertical eccentric viewing point.

67 56 47 33 68
346 863 972 33
4087 9365 2924
IT LA SO AM
LAP MAT PIN LIP
SIDE DESK SPIN
BETTER SLIDE

FIGURE 2-5 Large print (originally 72 point) reading training exercise showing capability of computer and laser or desk jet type printer to produce materials of nearly any desired size.

fingers may help to prevent losing one's place, and assist in locating the beginning of the next line.

Which devices to use for magnification during training

The Kraspegig used a high-powered COIL stand magnifier with a patterned mask and a custom window cut out.[24] The patient was to place the scotoma in the middle of the pattern and the window was cut to place the text in the best remaining vision.[24] The device demonstrated a good idea with the main flaw that it was tied to one magnifier, and that a horizontal eccentric viewing point was espoused. Jose is currently working on a theory that a peripheral dark ring acts as a peripheral lock of sorts, aiding eccentric viewing. Oddly enough, his favored practice magnifier is the old reliable high-powered COIL stand magnifier used in the Kraspegig.

There is no magical formula currently available to determine the optimal device to use during training. The devices that appear to achieve some success in the exam setting are a likely first choice, but the clinician must use his or her experience and assess the patient's motivation and frustration levels to determine if large print or other concessions might give the patient needed positive reinforcement in the early training stages.

Dealing with Patient Problems

Getting stuck—locking on the blind spot

It is important to reinforce with patients that they should not allow themselves to get stuck and frustrated on a single difficult word. The usual technique involves a two step process. First the patient should be encouraged to try to spell the word letter by letter; if that doesn't work then the patient should skip the word and move on. Often the patient can guess the word based upon the context, or the word may not be critical to understanding the paragraph. If the word turns out to be critical the patient can always go back to it later.

Errors of a consistent nature

Patients who consistently make similar mistakes may be routinely missing the beginning, end, or center of words, and filling in the missing letters by guesswork. Often, simple discussion of the problem is sufficient to begin the process of learning how to relocate the scotoma and avoid this problem.

Patient trying to read too fast

Most patients expect to read the same way they did before their eyes changed. They will often read very quickly, making numerous mistakes. It is helpful to remind patients that they need to begin more slowly and build speed slowly. One training option that is often helpful for these patients is to use lists of random words rather than meaningful text. The patient then must concentrate on each individual word rather than "skimming" for overall meaning.

Lack of comprehension

Patients frequently complain that they seem to be reading so slowly that they forget what they are reading about. It is important to reassure them that this is part of the learning process and that they should concentrate on the techniques now and not be concerned with comprehension, which will come later.

Headache/eyeache/dizziness

These symptoms are common and unavoidable. The patient should be warned that these will occur and that they are the result of muscular strain and tension and that reading will not harm the eyes. Failure to warn the patient could result in a major training setback. The patient should be instructed to take a break when these symptoms arise.

Fatigue

Just as with the previous symptoms, the patient is expected to fatigue more quickly than a normally sighted reader and certainly faster than the patient expects to fatigue. Numerous short practice sessions should be recommended rather than two or three long ones.

Frustration or lack of apparent motivation

When a patient, despite indications of solid goals, decides that it is too difficult or too much trouble to reach those goals, it is important to quickly discuss reassessing and lowering the goals, at least temporarily.

For example, the patient who wants to read books again for pleasure can be redirected to at least read for necessity (bills, mail, etc.) as a lower and hopefully temporary goal.

In-Office vs. Home Training

Cost

Clearly there is no comparison in cost to the patient when comparing in-office training with at-home training programs. Goodrich et al described a good in-office training program as requiring anywhere from 8 to 15 visits.[9] This is beyond the financial (as well as practical) reach of most of our elderly patients. Even if there were no fees for the training, the cost of transportation and time lost from work by accompanying family members would be too much to shoulder.

Success rates

This is an area where much research needs to be done. Little statistical data exist to show the relative effectiveness of one technique versus another, much less the efficacy of in-office training as compared to at-home training. There are many obvious benefits to in-office training. It is easier to monitor adherence to and correct application of any techniques and instructions, patient progress—or lack thereof—is easy to monitor, and midcourse corrections are easily made. On the other hand, there is often no way to ensure that compliance goes home with the patient, and the cost may create apprehension, unrealistic expectations, and cost-effectiveness arguments in the patient's mind. With at-home training patients are often on their own, but at least the training is free and patients must accept responsibility for their own efforts and success. They can still return periodically for follow-up, reinforcement, and midcourse corrections, but this may entail 2 to 4 additional visits rather than 8 to 15.

Need for research

While Goodrich and Quillman have demonstrated the success of in-office training techniques,[9] there has been little research to demonstrate which home training techniques, if any, are most successful.

The Future of Eccentric Viewing Training

Image Remapping

Much research is being done in this area with tremendous funding coming from NASA and the VA at this time. It remains to be seen whether remapping the image from the central area around the periphery of the central scotoma will help. The research indicating that most patients successfully locate a PRL seems to run counter to indications that this technique will be useful, but only actual testing will demonstrate its usefulness or lack thereof.

Scanning Laser Ophthalmoscope—In Assessment, Training, and Selecting EV Points

The scanning laser ophthalmoscope, used with its graphics capability, offers tremendous benefits in research and possible future training and rehabilitation efforts. Research with the SLO has already shown most of the standard functional field tests used in a low vision evaluation to be limited at best.

Using a scanning laser ophthalmoscope to test the validity of patients' Amsler grid responses showed Amsler grid reports to have poor validity. The instability of the PRL for fixation made mapping of the scotoma boundaries inaccurate. SLO studies have shown the adaptation to a PRL to be naturally developed by the visual system in response to a central scotoma. The PRL in these studies was not always the most light sensitive of the areas studied. They showed PRL selection tended to avoid having scotoma below fixation or to the left of fixation. Early SLO studies also demonstrated that the presence or absence of a central scotoma was a more powerful predictor of reading speed than visual acuity.[6]

Visual field accuracy without the SLO has no method of monitoring or compensating for retinal movement (even a blind spot monitoring technique allows for a 5 degree unsteadiness). An early SLO study showed that SLO scotoma maps were 3 to 30 degrees larger than tangent screen mapped scotomas, although overall shapes agreed well. PRL was found to be immediately adjacent to scotoma but not necessarily at the closest possible point to the fovea. Only sophisticated laboratory techniques like SLO and magnetic search coil techniques are capable of giving reliable maps of central scotomas.

CLINICAL PEARL

Only sophisticated laboratory techniques like SLO and magnetic search coil techniques are capable of giving reliable maps of central scotomas.

SLO is proposed as an answer to simplify training by helping to select a PRL that has optimal characteristics for reading, but it overlooks the tendency of the patient to select a PRL that may not be closest to the fovea, and it also ignores questions of stability (today's PRL may be tomorrow's scotoma). It may show us the reason a patient is having difficulty, often despite relatively good acuity, in cases where the PRL or even the fovea itself may be surrounded by scotomas, making continuous text reading very difficult (Figure 2-6). With the SLO, words and text can be placed on the patient's active or proposed PRL to assess the practicality of reading continuous text with that

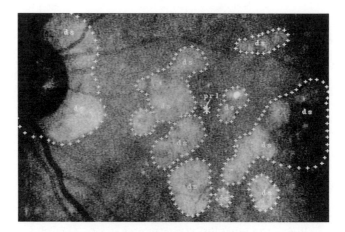

FIGURE 2-6 Scanning laser ophthalmoscope photograph showing dense scotomas (ds), and preferred retinal locus (PRL) marked by asterisk. Threshold scotomas may also be marked (ts) when present. This complex scotoma pattern contains many small dense scotomas that may not be perceived by the patient, and into which letters or parts of words may disappear when reading. (From Schuchard RA et al: *Clin Eye Vis Care* 6(3):103, 1994. Used with permission.)

point and to help begin training that point to use for reading (Figure 2-7). It can also be used to monitor if the PRL is being used successfully.

The approximately $100,000 cost of the SLO along with the expertise required to use it, and the time involved in doing the testing all render the instrument impractical for clinical use at the present time. Currently available software for the instrument may also limit its usefulness to the average doctor who is not well versed in programming. This should be a temporary problem only, as researchers are working to make the instrument easier to use and more versatile for the average clinician. In the meanwhile, the instrument is best used by regional referral centers where problem patients may be sent.

The assumption by researchers that accurate PRL and scotoma measurement are important for tasks like reading, face recognition, visual search, and spatial perception, may sound logical but appears to run contrary to clinical experience. Most low vision practitioners have been training patients successfully without this information. If SLO research shows us anything, it is that those practitioners who have been doing long tedious tests with the Amsler grid and tangent screen, thinking that they were doing a better job for their patients, may have been wasting their time. The fact that we have seen any success at all, may indicate that the appropriate training regimen may be successful for most patients without the need for expensive tests. In addition, we are all aware that any test, no matter how accurate, only represents a single moment in time. The very instability that is

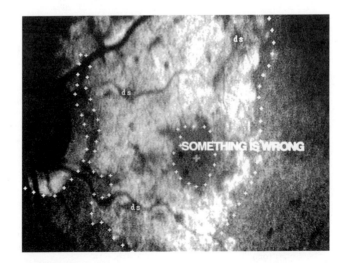

FIGURE 2-7 Scanning laser ophthalmoscope (SLO) photograph showing a simple sentence as read by the patient. The patient does not perceive the scotoma and thus misses the second part of the word "something" and the word "is". Theoretically the patient would read this as "some wrong". (From Schuchard RA et al: *Clin Eye Vis Care* 6(3):105, 1994. Used with permission.)

commonly seen means that even the best current test may have limited usefulness. That is not to say that the SLO has nothing to offer. The cases that we find as failures in clinical practice may be helped by having this more accurate information available. The void in research about what really happens in macular degeneration is finally beginning to be filled by work with this fascinating instrument.

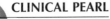

CLINICAL PEARL

The appropriate training regimen may be successful for most patients without the need for expensive tests.

CLINICAL PEARL

Any test, no matter how accurate, only represents a single moment in time.

References

1. Timberlake GT, Mainster MA, Peli E, et al: Reading with a macular scotoma, I. Retinal location of scotoma and fixation area, *Invest Ophthalmol Vis Sci* 27:1137-1147, 1986.
2. Wetter JJ, Wing GL, Trempe CL, Mainster MA: Visual acuity related to retinal distance from the fovea in macular disease, *Annals Ophthalmol* 16:174-176, 1982.

3. White JM, Bedell HE: The oculomotor reference in humans with bilateral macular disease, *Invest Ophthalmol Vis Sci* 31:1149–1161, 1990.
4. Legge GE, Ross JA, et al: Psychophysics of reading, clinical predictors of low-vision reading speed, *Invest Ophthal Vis Sci* 33:677-687, 1992.
5. Freeman PB: Personal communication, March 1995.
6. Fletcher DC, Schuchard RA: Scanning laser ophthalmoscope macular perimetry and applications for low vision rehabilitation clinicians, *Ophthalmol Clin North Am* 7(2):257-265, 1994.
7. Schuchard RA, Fletcher DC: Preferred retinal locus, a review with applications in low vision rehabilitation, *Ophth Clinica of North America* 7:243-256, 1994.
8. Griffen JR: *Binocular anomalies, procedures for vision therapy,* Chicago, 1976, Professional Press.
9. Goodrich GL, Quillman RD: Training eccentric viewing, *Vis Impair Blindness* 71:377-381, 1977.
10. Romayananda et al: Prismatic scanning method for improving visual acuity in patients with low vision, *Ophthalmology* 89:937-944, 1982.
11. Rosenberg R, Faye EE, Fischer M, Budick D: Role of prism relocation in improving visual performance of patients with macular dysfunction, *Opt Vis Science* 66(11):747-750, 1989.
12. Bailey I: Can prisms control eccentric viewing?, *Optom Monthly* 360-362, July 1983.
13. Kommerell G, Taumer R: Investigations of the eye tracking system through stabilized retinal images, *Bibl Ophthalmol* 82:288-297, 1972.
14. Peli E, Goldstein RB, Young GM, Trempe CL, Buzney SM: Image enhancement for the visually impaired, stimulations and experimental results, *Invest Ophthalmol Vis Sci* 32:2337-2350, 1991.
15. Freeman PB, Jose RT: *The art and practice of low vision,* Boston, 1991, Butterworth-Heinemann.
16. von Noorden GK, Mackensen G: Phenomenology of eccentric fixation, *Am J Ophthalmol* 53:642-661, 1962.
17. Goodrich GL, Mehr EB: Eccentric viewing training and low vision aids: current practice and implications of peripheral retinal research, *Am J Optom Physiol Opt* 63(2):119-126, 1986.
18. Cummings RW, Whittaker SG, Watson GR, Budd JM: Scanning characters and reading with a central scotoma, *Am J Optom Physiol Opt* 62(12):833-843, 1985.
19. Rubin GS: Vision and reading, *Ophthalmol Clin North Am* 7:237-241, 1994.
20. Whittaker SG, Budd J, Cummings RW: Eccentril fixation with macular scotoma, *Invest Ophthalmol Vis Sci* 29:268–278, 1988.
21. Holcomb JG, Goodrich GL: Eccentric viewing training, *J Am Optom Assoc* 47(11):1438-1443, 1976.
22. Peli E: Control of eye movement with peripheral vision: implications for training of eccentric viewing, *Am J Optom Physiol Opt* 63:113-118, 1986.
23. Goodrich GL: Personal communication, March 1995.
24. Epstein LI, Clarke AM, Hale RK, McNeer PR: A reading aid for patients with macular blindness, *Ophthalmologica* 183:101-104, 1981.

For additional information

Campbell, Ritter: *Clinical adaptation studies of the human retina:* Straatsma BR, Hall MO: *The retina: morphology, function and clinical characteristics,* 13-44, Berkeley, 1969, University of California Press.
Fridal G, Jansen L, Klindt M: Courses in reading development for partially sighted students, *Vis Impair Blindness* 1981.
Goodrich GL, Mehr EB, Overbury: Training materials to optimize residual vision, *Invest Ophthalmol Vis Sci* 26:219, 1985, SUPP.
Inde K: Low vision training in Sweden, *J Vis Impair Blindness* 72:307-310, 1978.

Maplesden C: A subjective approach to eccentric viewing training, *J Vis Impair Blindness* 78:5-6, 1984.

Quillman RD: *Low vision training manual,* Kalamazoo, 1980, Western Michigan University.

Schuchard RA: Validity and interpretation of Amsler grid reports, *Arch Ophthalmol* 111:776-780, 1993.

Schuchard RA, Fletcher DC, Maino JH: A scanning laser ophthalmoscope (SLO) low-vision rehabilitation system, *Clin Eye Vision Care* 6:101-107, 1994.

Timberlake GT, Peli E et al: Reading with a macular scotoma, II. Retinal locus for scanning text, *Invest Ophthalmol Vis Sci* 28:1268-1274, 1987.

3

Visual Impairment and Visual Efficiency Training

Brendal Waiss
Jay M. Cohen

Key Terms

visual rehabilitation	vision training	dynamic acuity
behavioral	low vision	accommodation
optometry	oculomotor skills	gross motor skills
visual therapy	binocularity	

In the field of low vision, the emphasis on "function" is foremost. Low vision practitioners will always try to avoid defining visual impairment in terms of absolute numerical values for acuities and/or visual fields. Instead, clinicians much prefer to speak in terms of the patient's abilities to function in the real world and what optical or nonoptical devices may be needed to increase the patient's ability to function. On a more sophisticated level, we should also think in terms of what visual skills the patient already possesses, which skills need improvement, and what skills can be taught to the patient to lead to enhanced function.

Historically one other visual specialty (that is, behavioral vision or vision training) employs the term function. Most of the time vision training caters to the pediatric population for binocular, accommodative, oculomotor/visual motor deficiencies, or perceptual problems.[1-3] Currently, vision therapy for adults is becoming more commonplace.[4,5] In addition, visual therapy for head trauma/stroke patients is being offered by some specialty practitioners.[6,7]

There seems to be a natural common bond between the rehabilitation treatment offered by low vision practitioners and the rehabilitative techniques of behavioral vision practitioners. It is only when the low vision practitioner incorporates vision therapy concepts into the treatment plan that comprehensive care is given.

In this brief chapter, it will be assumed that the reader accepts the fact that some type of visual efficiency training for low vision patients must take place both when the patient *is* using low vision devices and when he or she is *not* using any devices. In the circumstance when a device is used, it is assumed that the patient has been fully instructed by the practitioner or other designated personnel on the proper use and maintenance of any optical devices.[8,9] It is only after the patient is well-versed in the use of the devices that these "tools" can be incorporated into visual efficiency training. It is beyond the scope of this chapter to discuss how to best train patients in the correct use of their low vision devices or if indeed such training need be conducted by the practitioner or other designated personnel.

Many believe that congenitally visually impaired children can develop good temporal-spatial relationships of their visual world and can navigate and manipulate objects in the world as well as their motor/physical conditions permit. Many could argue that in caring for the congenitally visually impaired, visual efficiency training should be unnecessary because the patient will have had time to develop the abilities commensurate with his or her visual level through life experience and should be able to make full use of them. On the other hand, since the adventitiously visually impaired individual has had the opportunity to develop a normal primary visual direction, it is simply a matter of shifting visual direction after the central vision is impaired. We have found clinically that these two scenarios may not necessarily be true premises.

A simplistic view of low vision care is predicated on the idea that if all low vision patients could receive their appropriate low vision devices, mere possession would enable them to maximize their function. But possessing an actual device, and knowing how to use that device, is often not enough. Visual efficiency training is one area which has been virtually ignored and rarely offered to patients. The reasons to advocate for visual efficiency training would be: (1) to encourage eccentric viewing by establishing or reinforcing an eccentric pattern at distance and near after central vision is impaired (this is more fully addressed in Chapter 11 of this book), (2) to enhance binocular function (by increasing binocular ranges or eliminating diplopia), and (3) to improve scanning strategies to compensate for field defects. Ultimately when the patient's skills are up to par, there is an expected concomitant enhanced use of the prescribed low vision device.

CLINICAL PEARL

The reasons to advocate for visual efficiency training would be: (1) to encourage eccentric viewing (2) to enhance binocular function and (3) to improve scanning strategies.

We will present an overview of a possible assessment, training, and posttherapy assessment paradigm for practitioners who would like to begin to incorporate visual efficiency training into their low vision rehabilitation.

Assessment Testing of Patient's Abilities

To begin with, it is very important to observe as the patient navigates through your office. As you conduct the examination, listen to what the patient says about how he or she manages to compensate for the visual problem or tells you what their visual problems seem to be. Family members or significant others who accompany the patient to the exam may also provide insight into the coping mechanisms as well as the difficulties the patient is having. Other professionals' reports can also yield important information (Table 3-1).

We offer the following clinical paradigm to test major visual areas, over and beyond the usual low vision areas tested such as distance and near visual acuities, visual fields (peripheral and central), contrast sensitivity, and glare. We suggest a combined evaluation of what is more traditionally thought of as visual training areas such as oculo-motor skills (including fixations, saccades, and pursuits), gross and fine motor skills, speed and span of recognition (including visual memory), dynamic acuity abilities, and binocularity assessments.[10]

Even though in most cases low vision patients have limited binocu-larity, some patients perform best if they can retain their limited binocularity either through visual training, optical treatment via prism incorporation, or via biofeedback. The benefit to the patient of enhanced visual performance under binocular vision is sometimes too intangible for the doctor to prejudge based solely on clinical test results. Logic dictates that in cases of disparate acuities, visual fields,

TABLE 3-1

Limited Listing of Commonly Voiced Problems and Possible Areas to Investigate

Subjective complaint	Areas(s) to assess
Skips words/sentences, rereads lines/phrases	Central field, post stroke/trauma hemifield loss, ocular motility, binocularity problems (diplopia), accommodation problems, processing problem
Slow reading rate	Magnification too high, poor facility with low vision devices, field involvement, ocular motility/binocular problems, accommodation problems, processing problems
Word/letter reversals	Processing problem, laterality or directionality problem
Poor content retention of material read	Processing problem, poor use of devices, visual memory problem
Covers/closes one eye	Disparate acuities, contrast, fields, binocular status (diplopia)
Head turn/tilt or eccentric viewing	Central scotoma, binocularity problem, null point for nystagmus
Double vision	Binocular status (diplopia), disparate acuities, contrast, fields, high uncorrected astigmatism, refractive errors, media irregularities
Writes crooked	Interfering scotoma, poor motor skills, poor eye-hand coordination, binocular status
Copying errors	Interfering scotoma, poor motor skills, poor eye-hand coordination, binocular status, visual memory problem

or contrast, a clinical trial of occlusion of the poorer eye might improve the patient's visual function but ultimately, the patient's subjective responses should dictate whether the occlusion was beneficial, detrimental, or had no impact on performance and whether it should be part of the rehabilitation treatment plan.

CLINICAL PEARL

Even though in most cases low vision patients have limited binocularity, some patients perform best if they can retain their limited binocularity.

While occlusion at near point might be recommended, full time occlusion is discouraged because of its potential negative impact on real world activities such as mobility. Occlusion removes depth perception clues and reduces the peripheral visual field information contributed by the poorer eye. Full time occlusion might be recommended if there were intractable diplopia or such gross image distortion from the poorer eye that visual confusion was present.

CLINICAL PEARL

Full time occlusion might be recommended if there were intractable diplopia or such gross image distortion from the poorer eye that visual confusion was present.

Oculomotor Assessment

Asking patients to follow a moving target is a gross assessment of basic oculomotor motilities, tracking, pursuits, and rotations, but it can yield valuable information about the extent of eye movements for each eye as well as deviations in binocular/biocular conditions when in certain fields of gaze. The quality or smoothness of the movements can also be evaluated. Appropriately sized illuminated or nonilluminated targets should be used. The patient should be asked to follow the target with the eyes only. (When the task can only be achieved with gross head movement, it is important to note this.) The instructional set should be given first monocularly, then binocularly. The convergence of the eyes can also be monitored at this point when an accommodative target is used. Movements could be graded for accuracy and smoothness, and range of motion notations should be made.

For a finer assessment of fixations, appropriately enlarged standard tests used in vision training practice can be modified quite easily via photocopying enlargement or via laser printers, reprinting the materials in a size appropriate for patients. We have had experience with the commonly used tests such as the NYSOA King Devick or Developmental Eye Movement Test (DEM), and these may be considered. The Pepper Visual Skills Analysis Test can also be used.[11] With any pretest, remember not only to time the patient, but also to keep score of the number of errors and the type of errors made. In addition, some low vision texts have samples of reading tests that can be used.[12-14]

Binocular Fusion Assessment

Although the majority of our patients are not strabismic, most of our patients are not fully binocular. Surprisingly enough, many low vision patients suffer tremendously when their vergences cannot meet the demand placed on them because of the closer working distance common to low vision patients. We automatically assume that if the patient is given a stock prism reading prescription, then the patient will not put a strain on fusional abilities, but this is not the case. Younger people especially will hold the material closer than the calculated working distance because they can contribute their own accommodation. The patient's own vergence abilities may have been fragile to begin with so that the stock lens does not provide the amount the patient actually needs. (In that case it would be far better for the patient if the amount of required prism for fusion was actually measured and specifically fabricated into the glasses for the patient.)

Binocularity testing should be done both at distance and at near point. A very simple test which yields useful information is to shine a penlight toward the patient and view the position of the reflex relative to each eye to assess alignment. For both distance and near, when a large enough target is used, a quick cover test and prism bar or loose prisms can give valuable information. However, one must remember that the presence of a central scotoma will complicate interpretation of the results because it negates the need to precisely refixate after the cover test's occlusion, since the use of eccentric viewing points may have replaced the macula as the primary visual direction.

CLINICAL PEARL

One must remember that the presence of a central scotoma will complicate interpretation of the results because it negates the need to precisely refixate.

Other simple tests that we have successfully employed are the Convergence Near Point (CNP) test with an accommodative target, Brock string with large beads, Red Lens test, and Worth-4-dot. Large peripheral stereo targets (such as the Quoit Rings or large stereo animals) can be used to measure gross stereopsis for this population.

For some patients, more "sophisticated" binocular fusion tests cannot be administered. Simple comparisons of monocular versus binocular performance on tests such as acuities, Amsler grid, and contrast sensitivity testing can reveal how much assistance or interference exists. Remember to ask the patient for subjective impressions.

Accommodation Assessment

This is not usually a significant factor because children may have sufficient accommodative reserve for the demand and because many of our low vision patients are presbyopic. Furthermore since blur is a stimulus to accommodation, when there is loss of central vision, the feedback loop for regulating accommodation is compromised. In most cases, spectacles must be used because the need for high magnification requires amounts of plus impossible to generate through mere accommodation.

Obviously in prepresbyopes amplitudes and facilities can be assessed and will give more insight into the patient's ability to function.

Gross Motor Assessment

Most often only head trauma patients receive gross motor assessments by the occupational therapist or physical therapist involved with that particular person's case. Unfortunately, these assessments are not offered to most adventitious or congenital low vision patients. It is likely that most low vision patients may not need gross motor assessment but some could certainly benefit from more coordination skills.

CLINICAL PEARL

It is likely that most low vision patients may not need gross motor assessment but some could certainly benefit from more coordination skills.

The assessment begins when we watch the patient navigating the corridor, entering the exam room, and sitting down. Because our patients may have poor motor coordination as well as a visual problem, when doing gross motor assessments one needs to be aware of the patient's physical safety because the ability to detect and avoid common office obstacles may be reduced. Simple modifications can be made in the office such as padding any sharp corners and low hanging obstacles and putting tape on the floor as a pattern to be followed instead of using a raised walking rail.

Many techniques can be found in the materials produced by the Optometric Extension Program (OEP), College of Visual Development (COVD), or other books discussing vision training.[15,16]

We welcome the idea that at least now, children are given the opportunity to be involved in adaptive gym activities in schools so that they can develop improved skills in a supervised and safe setting.

Perceptual Assessments

Some practitioners are not comfortable administering perceptual assessments. However, these tests can yield valuable information especially when the visual impairment is secondary to the effects of head trauma or stroke. Some areas to consider for testing include visual memory, visual span, figure ground, figure constancy and spatial relationships, and visual perception. Further evaluation of factors such as laterality and left-right concepts can be evaluated using chalk board circles, Piaget left-right assessments and the peg board testing.[15,16] It is important to try to find some tests that do not depend on verbal or motor skills because these areas may be problematic to the patient.

Auditory Assessments

It is well known that many pathologies which adversely affect vision, also affect hearing. Even when the particular pathology only affects vision, an audiological evaluation is still important because one must know if hearing can be relied upon to help compensate for deficient visual cues.

Although we would like to assume that all children are evaluated somewhere along the way within the educational system, and that all adventitiously impaired patients get tested at some point in the rehabilitation process, this is not the case.

A brief auditory assessment for attention, discrimination, manipulation, or memory does not supplant a full workup by a speech pathologist/audiologist. Brief assessments can serve to prompt the patient or caretakers of the patient to act more quickly when a problem is discovered.

General Considerations for Visual Efficiency Training

It is best to sequence and organize all training so that the patient will not only learn the specific training technique but also integrate the underlying skill and transfer it into daily living activities both with and without the use of the low vision devices. Training can be very frustrating so it is helpful to devise small stepwise incremental goals in training, and seek activities where the patient can find and easily monitor his or her own success. In order to avoid fatiguing the patient, do not make the training session too long.

CLINICAL PEARL

Sequence and organize all training so that the patient will not only learn the specific training technique but also integrate the underlying skill and transfer it into daily living activities.

Easily understood techniques should be given to the patients so that they can practice at home. Some patients may be too nervous or perhaps are unable to cognitively absorb in-office instruction efficiently. Whenever possible, involve family members or significant others in the process. Giving the patient and family members customized written or computer printed/produced instructional sets can be very beneficial. Providing a written instructional set emphasizes the importance of doing the exercises and reduces the patient's apprehension about performing them correctly.

Visual Efficiency Training

There is no shortage of training exercises for each of the areas we touched upon: oculomotor skills, binocularity, accommodative, and even gross motor. The only thing which needs to be remembered is that actual training of skills is akin to amblyopia therapy in that it requires the use of enlarged targets appropriate to the patient's acuity, closer than usual working distances, high contrast training materials, eccentric viewing training, and eventually incorporation of the appropriate low vision device into this training regimen. This can be accomplished by enlarging material via photocopying or by enlarging the font of some printers. Some training materials can be produced as overheads or slides. These projected materials can easily be enlarged by moving the projector further from the screen and then refocusing the materials, or by having the patient sit closer to or further from the screen. These activities are great because they are done in free space.

> **CLINICAL PEARL**
> *Actual training of skills requires the use of enlarged targets closer than usual working distances, high contrast training materials, eccentric viewing training, and incorporation of the appropriate low vision device.*

Visual efficiency training for low vision patients also requires an area in the office where additional task lighting can be provided and where posture improving tilt tables are available for working with near point materials.

Hemianopia Training

Hemianopia training is a special type of training because most frequently those patients have been assessed by occupational and physical therapists for gross motor training but generally are not counseled on the visual remediation available. It is incumbent upon the clinician to introduce compensating devices to the patient such as mirrors and prisms. If the patient accepts these devices, training should incorporate their use. In many cases, the patient may reject the prism or the mirror, but the clinician should make the patient aware of various scanning strategies such as head or eye movement scanning. Often in the beginning, especially if there is neglect involved, auditory feedback or tactile feedback can be of assistance as a "gentle" reminder.

Posttraining Assessments

In order to more seriously monitor the patient's progress, one must do pretraining skills assessment, conduct a training program, and follow up with a posttraining assessment. It is important to ask the patient or significant other to subjectively report if any improvements have been observed since therapy was initiated. The practitioners should also objectively measure progress in these areas. One should avoid using the same "testing" materials as "training" materials. There are enough different ways to measure the extent of the skill so that there can be a difference in testing versus training materials.

Conclusion

More than the standard battery of typical low vision tests should be considered for our low vision patients. While many other disciplines or professions are now stating that they too can provide low vision care on par with the optometric low vision practitioner, we believe that optometrists, with their unique educational background and orientation to provide functional vision care, render the best possible service and make optometric low vision services unique.

The best model of comprehensive low vision care is the multidisciplinary approach where the professionals offer the patient their full scope of services, conferencing their findings with each other, the patient, and significant others; and then provide coordinated services with the patient's best interest taking precedence.

References

1. Ludlum W, Kleinman BI: The long range results of orthoptic treatment of strabismus, *Am J Optom Arch Am Acad Optom* 42(11):647-684, 1965.
2. Hoffman L, Cohen AH: Effectiveness of non-strabismic optometric vision training in a private practice, *Am J Optom Arch Am Acad Optom* 50(10):813-816, 1973.
3. Greenstein TN (ed): *Vision and learning disability,* St Louis, 1976, American Optometric Association.
4. Morton D: A pilot project to study the effects of enhancing visual function, visual guided mobility, and visually guided coordination on independence in the elderly, *J Optom Vis Dev* 15(4):23-26, 1984.
5. *Vision therapy news backgrounder,* St Louis, 1985, American Optometric Association.
6. Cohen AH, Soden R: An optometric approach to the rehabilitation of the stroke patient, *J Am Optom Asso* 52(10):795-800, 1981.
7. Fowler MS, Richardson MA, Stein JF: Orthoptic investigation of neurological patients undergoing rehabilitation, *Br Orthopt J* 48:2-7, 1991.
8. Goodlaw EI: Homework for low vision patients, *Am J Optom Arch Am Acad Optom* 45(8):532-538, 1968.
9. Goodrich GL, Mehr EB, Quillman RD, Shaw HK, Wiley JK: Training and practice effects in performance with low vision aids: a preliminary study, *Am J Optom Arch Am Acad Optom* 54(5):312-318, 1977.
10. Hoffman L, Waiss B: Functionally based evaluation for low vision patients, *J Beh Optom* 1(5):127-129, 1990.
11. Freeman PB, Jose RT: *The art and practice of low vision,* Boston, 1991, Wail-Heinemann.
12. Backman O, Inde K: *Low vision training,* Malmo, 1979, LiberHermonds.

13. Quillman RD: *Low vision training manual,* Kalamazoo, 1980, Western Michigan University.
14. Jose R: *Understanding low vision,* New York, 1983, American Foundation for the Blind.
15. Suchoff I: *Visual-spatial development in the child: an optometric theoretical and clinical approach,* New York, 1974, SUNY State College of Optometry.
16. Groffman S, Solan H: *Developmental and perceptual assessment of learning disabled children: theoretical concepts and diagnostic testing,* Santa Ana, 1994, Optometric Extension Program.

Appendix 1: Resource List

Bernell
(full range of vision therapy testing/
    training equipment)
750 Lincolnway East
P.O. Box 4637
Southbend, IN 46634-4637
(800) 348-2225

College of Optometrists in Vision
    Development
    (information on vision therapy)
P.O. Box 285
Chula Vista, CA 92012

OPIS Communication Software
(customized patient communication
    software: low vision and
    vision therapy)
P.O. Box 1412
South Dennis, MA 02660
(800) 272-6747

Optometric Education Program
(vision therapy books, testing
    and training equipment)
2912 South Daimler Street
Santa Ana, CA 92705-5811

4

Functional Adaptive Devices

Douglas R. Williams

Key Terms

adaptive devices	reading stands	sensory substitution
relative size devices	writing devices	devices
large print	medical assistive	auditory
lighting control	devices	substitution
illumination control	mobility devices	tactile substitution
filters	canes	braille
posture and	dog guides	vision substitution
positioning	ETAs	
devices		

The successful prescribing, use of, and adaptation to many low vision devices depends on multiple factors. Among these factors is the acceptance of the device as being practical and functional for the patient. Adaptive devices can help achieve both these goals. Sometimes called nonoptical devices, these devices are commonly encountered by patients. However, they are rarely thought of as "prescriptive devices" or as being associated with the low vision prescribing process so they are often overlooked by both the practitioner and the patient. These devices can often be prescribed by themselves or used in conjunction with low vision optical devices to enhance function.

71

Adaptive devices can be grouped according to how their primary effects are produced. (See box below.)

Adaptive Low Vision Devices

Relative size devices
Light and illumination controls
Posture and positioning devices
Writing and communication devices
Medical assistive devices
Mobility assistive devices
Sensory substitution devices

CLINICAL PEARL

Adaptive devices can help achieve acceptance of low vision devices as being both practical and functional for the patient.

CLINICAL PEARL

Adaptive devices can be grouped according to how their primary effects are produced.

Relative Size Devices

Patients will often state that they can only see the large print in the newspaper or only read the headlines and not the standard newsprint. It is also very common for patients with low vision to read only the largest optotypes on the visual acuity chart and fail to read the smaller optotypes. These common occurrences attest to the value of larger print and are examples of relative size magnification. By far the most common adaptive devices are relative size devices. Relative size magnification simply involves making an object larger without changing its distance from the eye and without the use of lenses. The amount of magnification is a ratio of the original size object to that of the "enlarged" object. The angular size of the objects can be compared or the difference in size noted and the amount of magnification determined by direct measurement. When the original, or standard object is not readily available, sometimes the amount of magnification is difficult to determine. The standard for normal-size print is approximately 10 point; thus if print larger than 10 point is used, the magnification can be easily determined by dividing 10 into the size of the larger print. For example, 24 point type will produce 2.4X magnification relative to 10 point type.

> **CLINICAL PEARL**
>
> *By far the most common adaptive devices are relative size devices.*

Large Print

Large print is by far the most common relative size adaptive device. The concept of what constitutes large print in typography considers all the needs of the low vision patient. Besides the size of the print, there are the factors relating to the darkness of the print, inking characteristics, weight and color of the paper, spacing of the letters, spacing between lines, size of margins, and the type style. Large print materials are usually produced with heavy leading, or wide spacing between the letters and lines of print; with a bold, simple, sans serif type style, and printed on a nonglossy paper that provides for good contrast and prevents glare. The Lighthouse Inc. has guidelines for print legibility with partial sight. Contrast, color, point size, leading, font style, font selection, letter spacing, margins, paper finish, and color are discussed in terms of improving legibility. Prince[1] outlined the desirable characteristics of large print to enhance legibility for the low vision reader:

1. The print should have clean edges.
2. The print should be of such a size that the lower case "o" will approximate 2.7 mm or more in the vertical direction. The strokes should not be too bold—not more than 17.5% of the letter height. These dimensions favor 18 point type.
3. The paper should have high contrast and good opacity. It should also be lightweight.
4. The line length should not be less than 36 picas (6 inches) in length.
5. Periods and commas should, if possible, be larger than those traditionally used. The period should be approximately 30% of the height of the lower case "o," and the comma should be approximately 55% of the lower case "o".
6. Hyphenation should be kept to a minimum, preferably eliminated entirely.

> **CLINICAL PEARL**
>
> *Large print is by far the most common relative size adaptive device.*

From a practical point of view, large print is limited in the amount of magnification that can be offered. Magnification is generally limited to approximately 2.4X. Fonda[2] has pointed out that large print is often used when standard print could be read if held at a closer distance, perhaps with the aid of lenses. Large print is also limited in availability. Many patients will have difficulty finding the material they want to read immediately available in large print. Additionally the added expense and space required for printing becomes a problem. When a special edition is printed in large print, the area required for the book is increased by the square of the magnification. Many single volume works become multiple volumes when converted to large print. Because of the simplicity of the large print, some partially-sighted patients may resist learning to use other types of magnifying devices.

Despite these obvious problems, there are some useful advantages to large print. The additional contrast provided by large print makes for improved reading performance in patients with contrast sensitivity problems. The large print allows the low vision patient to read by changes in size, spatial frequency, and additional contrast.

Large print may be useful in prescribing lower-powered optical systems where the development of reading and scanning skills is easier with lower optical magnification. Once these skills have advanced to allow easy reading and scanning, the use of smaller print combined with a higher-powered optical device may be in order to allow greater accessibility to a broader range of material. Early exposure and training with both magnifying and optical aids usually overcome the complete dependence upon large print or the problems encountered with nonadaptation to high-power optical systems.

CLINICAL PEARL

Large print may be useful in prescribing lower-powered optical systems where the development of reading and scanning skills is easier with lower optical magnification.

Large print books are available from many sources. Large print book publishers print books in both paperback and hardcover, and cater to a wide diversity of interests. Popular periodicals in large print include the *Reader's Digest*, the *New York Times*, and the *World at Large* (Figure 4-1). A limited selection of some other periodicals may be available in large print format. Additional source information can be found through the National Library Service for the Blind and Physically Handicapped (NLS). Large print is available for dictionaries, atlases, thesauri, cookbooks, and Bibles (Figure 4-2). *Large-Print Scores and Books Catalogue* is a guide to the large print collection in the music section of the NLS. The minimum type size is 14 point and the music staff is approximately 1 inch.

Large print typewriters and computers

Large print can also be produced using large print typewriters. Although the computer word processor has largely replaced the typewriter, the use of the typewriter for personal communication should not be overlooked. There is still a large population of visually impaired individuals who may also be intimidated by computer technology and would find the typewriter a more acceptable and cost effective alternative. The typewriter still offers a convenient way for the low vision patient to communicate. Developing typing skills can be valuable in maintaining communication with others. The specifications for large type produced by a typewriter differ somewhat from that used in print typography.

The size of typewriter print is designated by the term *pitch*. The pitch is a unit used to measure the number of typewritten characters per horizontal inch. Thus 6 pitch type would have six typewritten characters per horizontal inch. The smaller the pitch, the larger the type size. The term *pitch* by itself, however, does not indicate the vertical dimension of the type size.

Standard typewriters usually have either pica type, measuring 10 pitch or 10 letters to the horizontal inch; or elite type, measuring 12 pitch or 12 letters to the horizontal inch. Most manufacturers specify only pitch and not the point size of the type styles available. With large print typewriters, the number of single line spaces per vertical inch can vary considerably. The National Braille Association considers 3 single space lines per vertical inch to be the maximum acceptable for large print typewriters. In order for the print to be considered "large print," it has been recommended that the lower case letters measure at least $\frac{1}{8}$ inch to approximate 18 point print.

Computer access for the low vision patient has created a need for large print software. Several onscreen programs will produce large print text and graphics on both IBM- and Macintosh-compatible computers. A distinct advantage in using large print software is that the font of the print can be selected to fit the needs of the viewer. Some large print access for the computer does not always involve stand-alone software. Some programs and access involve having a specific type of computer board installed. When dealing with large print computer access software, it is desirable to have "silent software." Once loaded into the memory of the computer, silent software will enlarge whatever program the viewer is using without interfering with that program. In addition to the software that is currently

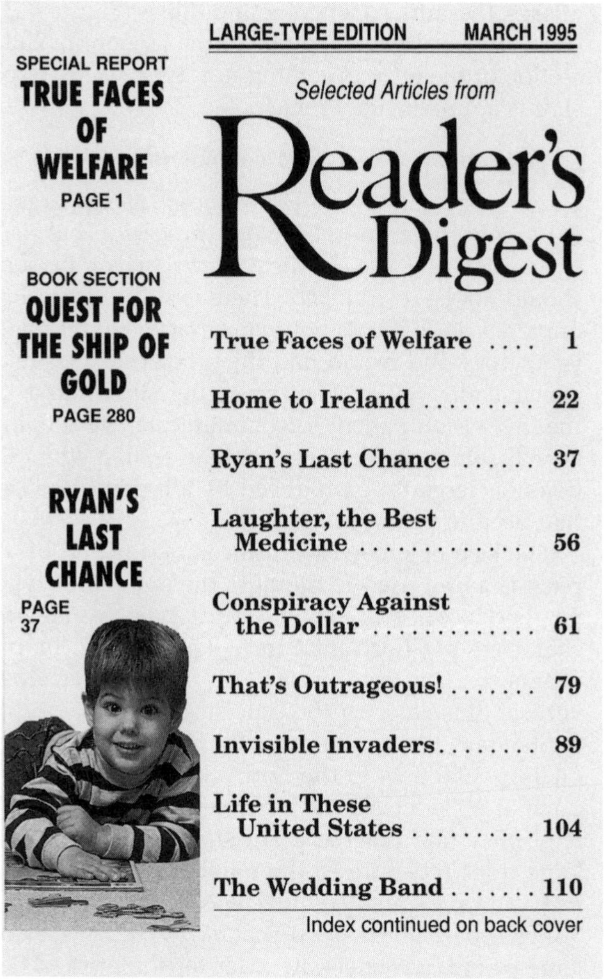

LARGE-TYPE EDITION MARCH 1995

SPECIAL REPORT
TRUE FACES OF WELFARE
PAGE 1

Selected Articles from
Reader's Digest

BOOK SECTION
QUEST FOR THE SHIP OF GOLD
PAGE 280

RYAN'S LAST CHANCE
PAGE 37

True Faces of Welfare 1
Home to Ireland 22
Ryan's Last Chance 37
Laughter, the Best Medicine 56
Conspiracy Against the Dollar 61
That's Outrageous! 79
Invisible Invaders........ 89
Life in These United States 104
The Wedding Band 110

Index continued on back cover

FIGURE 4-1 Large print *Reader's Digest* compared to the standard edition. The 18 point type of the large print edition of *Reader's Digest* will provide 2.0X relative size magnification compared to the 9 point type of the standard edition. *Continued*

available, full page monitors are available that provide for enlarged output. Caution should be exercised in that some graphic-oriented programs are not compatible with some computer enlargement programs. Zoomtext Plus and Vista are two IBM-compatible programs with the capacity to enlarge graphics.

Other Relative Size Devices

Being able to manage one's personal financial affairs is important for almost everyone. Writing checks and balancing a checkbook are basic

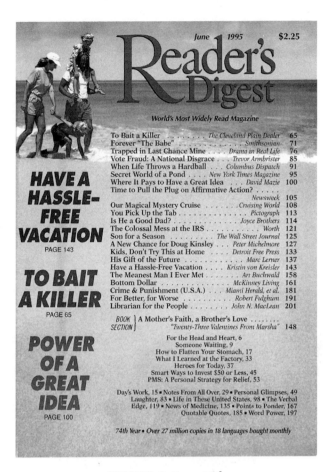

FIGURE 4-1, cont'd.

elements in personal financial management. Large print checks with a format of raised and embossed bold lines make this job easier. Deluxe Check Printers distributes a special format business-size check suitable for many low vision patients. The check style, called the Guideline, is available through most banking institutions (Figure 4-3). The check register is also included in a large, boldface format making entries easier to see.

The telephone is a vital communication link, especially for the visually impaired who often rely upon it to carry out their daily activities. The task of dialing a phone can be troublesome for some patients if they must see the small letters or numerals on the instrument. Large print overlays for both rotary and push button phones are available from a variety of sources. Caution must be exercised because most of these overlays have enlarged numbers, but the letters on the dial are either missing or lack any enlargement.

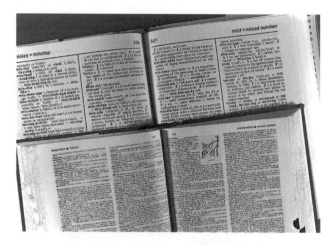

FIGURE 4-2 Large print Webster's dictionary compared to the standard edition. The large print edition uses a larger size for each page. (From Merriam-Webster's New Collegiate Dictionary, by Merriam-Webster Inc. Used with permission.)

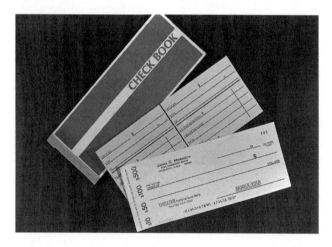

FIGURE 4-3 Large print checks. The Guideline by Deluxe Check Printers offers large print checks and large print deposit tickets as well as a large print check register.

Voice activated or automatic dial phones can assist with this problem. Big button phones are available from several distributors (Figure 4-4). Large-face quartz watches make the task of telling time easier. Faces are available in either white face with black hands and numbers, or reverse contrast—black face with white hands and numbers. Various styles have extra thick hands and numbers that are approximately $\frac{1}{4}$ inch high. Clocks and watches may be analog (hour and minute hand format) or digital format. The digital format is available in the "flip," light emitting diode (LED), or liquid crystal display (LCD). The flip

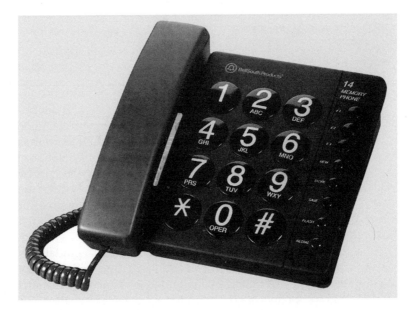

FIGURE 4-4 Large button phone. Note that although the numbers are large, the letters are printed smaller and may still be difficult to see. (Photo courtesy of The Lighthouse Inc.)

format uses high contrast numbers that flip as the time changes. The LCD format rarely provides the needed contrast and should be recommended with caution.

For recreation and pleasure, various games are available in large print editions. Scrabble, chess, checkers, backgammon, bingo, and many types of playing cards are some examples. Playing cards have various designs from large pips to letters and numbers up to 2 inches in size.

Sewing is an activity that many low vision patients curtail because of their eyesight. Spread eye needles are easy to thread and all sizes of thread and yarn can be used. Automatic needle threaders for both machine and hand sewing automatically handle this visually demanding task. Large print designs are available for embroidery. When measuring fabric, large type tape measures can be easily seen. Large head pins, colored pins, and magnetic pin holders ease the handling of pins. Colored beads provide the contrast necessary to see the pin against the pin cushion or fabric.

Lighting and Illumination Controls

Besides magnification, one of the major areas where assistance can be given to many low vision patients is that of accessory contrast control devices. The control of lighting and contrast sometimes can make the difference between performing a particular task or giving up.

![sphere icon] **CLINICAL PEARL**

Besides magnification, one of the major areas where assistance can be given to many low vision patients is that of accessory contrast control devices.

Johnston[3] has provided a diagrammatic representation of the contrast sensitivity function delineating a domain of contrast and object size (spatial frequency) (Figure 4-5). This representation clearly shows that with a change in contrast, an object can be moved from "nonseeing" to "seeing." Our current understanding of ocular disease has led to the concept that the retinal receptors are not simply functional to one spatial frequency, but rather function at many spatial frequencies and intensities of stimuli.

The type of ocular pathology will serve as a guideline to the type of functional vision loss to be anticipated, and will also serve somewhat as a suggested management guideline to restore function. Photophobia and complaints of glare are often experienced in patients with cataracts, early macular degeneration, albinism, and early diabetic retinopathy.

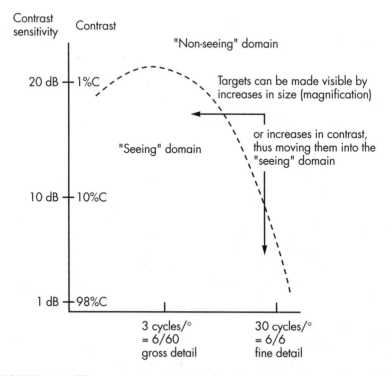

FIGURE 4-5 The contrast sensitiviy function delineates a "domain" of contrast and object size (spatial frequency) in which objects are visible. (Reproduced by permission of J. P. Lippincott Company.)

Severe photophobia is often encountered in achromatopsia, cone dystrophies, aphakia, and retinitis pigmentosa. With the loss of central vision, there is a need for higher illumination levels. The fact that the retinal receptors respond to more than one frequency and intensity often accounts for the seemingly different responses to lighting, contrast, and magnification. Retinitis pigmentosa patients with subcapsular cataracts should consider cataract extraction when the cataract limits functioning. Glaucoma patients who may be on miotics may be sensitive to outdoor glare or dim lighting indoors. Miotic fixed pupils can create a relatively dark adapted state and lower visual functioning when rod function is impaired. Advanced glaucoma often sees large nerve fiber layer damage so extensive that magnification is not useful. The contrast sensitivity function may well be below normal expecteds and improving contrast with filters will often help. Laser photocoagulation for diabetic retinopathy, which reduces night vision and contrast, may require special attention in these areas.

CLINICAL PEARL

The type of ocular pathology will serve as a guideline to the type of functional vision loss to be anticipated, and will also serve somewhat as a suggested management guideline to restore function.

Glare may cause discomfort or an uncomfortable sensation, and interfere with optimal vision. The glare that causes discomfort is termed *discomfort glare*, whereas glare that interferes with vision is termed *disability glare*. Glare sensitivity increases with normal aging and is often the result of ocular pathology. Although it is often difficult to evaluate the various factors contributing to a glare phenomenon, certain factors have been identified. The brightness of the source is important. In general the brighter the source, the greater the discomfort and interference with vision. By controlling the brightness with filters, the glare can be controlled. The size of the source is another factor. This is usually expressed in terms of the angle subtended at the eye. The larger the source, the greater the potential for creating glare. A large area of low brightness, however, may be as disturbing as a smaller source of higher brightness. The position of the source of light is another factor. Glare is reduced as the source is moved away from the line of sight. Contrast also plays a role in determining glare. The greater the contrast between the source and its surroundings, the greater will be the glare. Lastly, time is an important factor in glare. The longer a source is viewed, the greater will be the potential for the source to be glare producing. A source that is not disturbing for an exposure of a few minutes may become uncomfortable and fatiguing when a patient is exposed to it for an extended period of time.

Consideration in the selection of lighting can help reduce glare and control contrast to give optimum visual performance. Several types of lighting are now available for patient use. Fluorescent, incandescent, full-spectrum, halogen, neodymium, and various high-intensity light sources are available. Increased visual function can often be achieved for the low vision patient by appropriate selection and counseling about lighting.

CLINICAL PEARL

Consideration in the selection of lighting can help reduce glare and control contrast to give optimum visual performance.

Sunlight or daylight is often preferred by the visually impaired. Because it is natural, no problems exist with its cost and it is not considered to be harsh. Its control, however, can be a problem. At noon on a clear day with the sundirectly overhead, as high as 10,000 foot-candles may be available on a horizontal plane. Clear sky alone can provide more than 1500 footcandles and a clouded sky can provide as much as 4000 footcandles of illumination. Either outdoors or indoors, this illumination is not controllable and is often excessive. Slow light- and dark-adaptation, characteristically found in many low vision patients, can present a problem with daylight. A sudden shift of brightness can cause discomfort when adaptation cannot take place fast enough. Diffused sunlight can help reduce some of the problems of sunlight. Outdoor patios and porches can have covers that diffuse light, and indoor blinds and curtains that do not cut out light but diffuse it are recommended.

Fluorescent lighting often presents problems for many low vision patients. Fluorescent lights provide little contrast, because of the even lighting. Fewer shadows result with low contrast; however, the light is often perceived as harsh and tends to accentuate the blues, greens, and yellows. With fluorescence of the crystalline lens due to ultraviolet, there is often a haze or veiled glare associated with fluorescent lighting. The various "white" fluorescent lights now available make it possible to choose a "cool" or "warm" light for a given application. Fluorescent light is useful in that it is cooler. When prescribing lighting to be used with an optical device close to the eye, this can be an important factor.

Incandescent lighting (sometimes called filament lighting) has its main spectral output in the yellow portion of the spectrum. Incandescent lamps are more directional and the sources tend to be more pinpoint. In contrast to fluorescent lighting, incandescent lighting provides more contrast and thus is capable of producing more shadows. To solve some of these problems, shading that diffuses the light source can be used. Large reflector shades with diffusers are a very good source of illumination for many low vision applications. The small high-intensity lamps are excellent choices for work within a small area. The patient can move and position the light for the best effect. Incandescent light may be preferred by patients who have cataracts and other medial opacities. There is less scattering of the longer wavelengths from the spectral output of the lamp.

Neodymium light sources, marketed as Chromalux bulbs, may be useful for some patients. Available in 60 watt and 100 watt frosted bulbs, they provide for illumination which approaches sunlight and have been shown to improve reading performance on short term tasks when compared to incandescent illumination.

Halogen lighting has become popular with many patients. However, concern has been raised about ultraviolet output and the (erythematous) skin effects with increasing exposure to this type of light. The literature is scant with respect to the phototoxic ocular effects of halogen lighting in particular, but is abundant in ocular reports of the hazards and phototoxicity of ultraviolet exposure. Until additional and specific research is conducted, caution should be exercised with halogen lighting.

In addition to the various types of light, the light source can be controlled with the use of a rheostat. Unfortunately, there are few lamps available with the rheostat as part of the light itself. Instead, a separate rheostat may be used to control the illumination source by plugging the source into the variable control. These rheostats are more commonly designed for use with incandescent lighting sources than with fluorescent sources due to the nature of the electrical requirements for operating the lamps. Eschenbach now supplies some of its illuminated stand magnifiers with a variable halogen light source with a rheostat for adjustable brightness.

Filters

Filters can help control glare and improve function for many tasks. The various lens parameters that may be incorporated into the filter should be given consideration. Lens color, optical density, photochromaticity, polarization, selective band filters, UV coatings, and mirror coatings are factors to consider when selecting a filter.

CLINICAL PEARL

Lens color, optical density, photochromacity, polarization, selective band filters, UV coatings, and mirror coatings are factors to consider when selecting a filter.

Colored filters are designed to have specific characteristics of transmission through all portions of the spectrum. Caution should be used to ensure that a filter is not chosen solely upon color alone. In discussing glass absorptive filters, Borish[4] points out that the color of an absorptive lens is not a major factor, but merely a result of the colorant used. The most practical colors for the filter are those that offer the best visual acuity without loss of color perception. Protection from the adjacent spectral ultraviolet and infrared radiation is also important. The eye is not equally sensitive to all portions of the visual spectrum. The maximum sensitivity in a normal eye occurs under photopic conditions around 550 nm in the yellow-green while under photopic conditions shifts to the shorter wavelength of approximately 500 nm in the blue-green. This shift may be an important consideration when dealing with low vision patients who may have either a rod or cone dystrophy or other condition altering their peak sensitivity. Green lenses typically filter the colors of the spectrum so that the transmission curve matches that of the photopic sensitivity curve of the normal observer. Thus color perception should be affected very little. Neutral gray colored filters lower the transmission uniformly across the spectrum so that there is no color distortion. Amber or yellow filters are mainly designed to increase contrast by filtering out the shorter blue light which is more easily scattered. Unfortunately, many of the colored glass filters which enjoyed popularity in the past either have limited production and availability, or are not being manufactured at all. Tinted plastic has replaced many of these past trademark filters.

Optical density is a measure of the transmittance of a filter. The optical density is equal to the logarithm of the reciprocal of the transmittance. The higher the optical density, the lower is the transmittance of the filter. Shade numbers are occasionally used in place of optical density. The optical density is equal to $\frac{3}{7}$ (shade number −1). Table 4-1 lists the relationship between shade numbers, optical density, and transmittance.

Polarization can be used in filters to reduce glare. Much of what we see depends upon light reflected from objects. Nonpolarized filters can reduce the intensity of the source and thus help in the reduction of glare; however, these nonpolarized lenses have little effect on reflected light causing glare. Today polarized filters use an H-sheet Polaroid material developed in 1938 and are available in a wide variety of forms. These include both glass laminate and molded polarized CR-39 plastic in Plano, finished and semifinished single vision, bifocal, trifocal, and even progressive lens forms. The polarized lenses are available in many colors, including photochromatic materials, and even with the capability of being tinted.

Many of the filters that are in common use today were developed from the research that has been carried on by several investigators.[5-9]

TABLE 4-1
Relationship of Shade Number, Optical Density, and Transmittance

Shade number	Optical density	Transmittance %
1.0	0	100.00%
1.5	.214	61.10
1.7	.300	50.10
2.0	.429	37.30
2.5	.643	22.80
3.0	.857	13.90
4.0	1.286	5.18
5.0	1.714	1.93
6.0	2.143	0.72
7.0	2.571	0.27
8.0	3.000	0.10

Berson[9] suggested that an occluder be used to prevent light from reaching the retina in one eye in patients with retinitis pigmentosa. It was suggested that the occluded eye be kept "in reserve" for use when the other eye had deteriorated below a functional level. This theory grew out of a study on animal models where the damaging effects of general illumination on the retinal tissue were summarized as follows:

1. Normal retinas are more resistant to photic damage than degenerating retinas.
2. The damaging effect depends upon the intensity and duration of the illumination and also on the recovery period.
3. A sudden change from darkness to continuous bright light is particularly damaging.
4. The higher the body temperature above normal, the shorter the time required for the light of a given intensity to produce a damaging effect.
5. Light of equal energy but different spectral composition can damage the normal rat retina corresponding to its bleaching effect on visual purple (Rhodopsin).

Berson's occlusion was performed with a tightly fitting scleral lens. Unfortunately, the results showed that the occluded eye deteriorated just as fast as the nonoccluded eye. Further study did, however, suggest that if it was possible for light to be prevented from reaching the deteriorating rod segments, while still permitting enough light to enter the eye to be useful for cone functioning, the deterioration of the rod mechanism may be slowed. It was theorized that this could be done by using a filter whose absorption spectrum is closely matched by the action spectrum of rhodopsin. Since the main sensitivity of the cones is at a longer wavelength than that of the rods (555 nm vs.

507 nm), a filter matched to the rod sensitivity should allow sufficient light to enter the eye to activate the cones without markedly stimulating the rods to shed their outer segments. Adrian et al.[10] proposed that a filter to protect the retina from possible illumination damage have the following properties:

1. Low total light transmittance. It has been suggested that the filter have approximately 10% transmission outdoors and a higher transmission indoors.
2. The filter characteristics should protect the rods to a greater extent than the cones. That is, the cone-to-rod stimulation ratio (R) should be as high as compatible with useful vision.
   - Light having an equal energy spectrum, and neutral grey filters transilluminated by that light, have ratios of 1.0.
   - A blue filter, which preferentially transmits short wavelengths, has a ratio less than 1.0. The wavelengths transmitted are those to which the rods are particularly sensitive.
   - Filters that transmit mainly long visible wavelengths have ratios above 1.0. The cones are particularly sensitive to those wavelengths.
   - The latter filters (R greater than 1.0) have a reddish appearance, and at low transmittance levels are the ones desired for protection in retinitis pigmentosa.
3. The reduction of color discrimination through the filter should be as minimal as possible. At the very least, the filter should permit the identification of traffic lights, even by pedestrians.

Corning Glass Works proposed to develop such a filter for the retinitis pigmentosa patient, and the result was the CPF 550 lens.

Corning CPF filters

The Corning CPF 550 lens grew out of the search to find a lens with properties similar to the Adrian lens. Corning researchers found that the technology of photochromic features available in lens offered patients not only short wavelength attenuation, but also the capacity for the filter to darken in bright illumination and clear in darker illumination. The CPF filters combine the features of short wavelength filtering, photochromaticity, and the capability of prescription incorporation to create filters with a broad range of applications to many light sensitive patients. The special filtering of the CPF 550 lens is due to a special proprietary process in which a Photogrey Extra lens is surfaced and edged and then subjected to a high temperature hydrogen diffusion process which alters the absorption of the glass near the ocular surface. This color layer is less than .2 mm thick and produces the unique spectral absorption characteristics of the filter. The nonocular surface of the lens is then resurfaced so that the tint remains only in the ocular surface. The CPF 550, introduced in 1981, was the original lens in the CPF series and continues as the choice for patients who have intense sensitivity to light and poor dark-adaptation.

Patients with retinitis pigmentosa often select the CPF 550 lens as a lens of first choice. After the introduction of the CPF 550 filter, a lighter filter was sought for those patients who preferred higher levels of transmittance due to less severe symptoms. In 1983 Corning introduced the CPF 511 and CPF 527 filters. These lighter filters are used extensively by the majority of low vision patients but find particular usefulness for aphakes, pseudoaphakes, and patients with developing cataracts. Both lenses darken to brown in sunlight.

In 1989 Corning introduced its Design Series coating to add to the acceptance of these filters. The Design coating is applied to the CPF 527 and CPF 511 filters in a subtle, multiple-layer mirror coating. The special mirror coating adds an antireflection feature and a flash mirror to enhance reflection. The spectral cutoffs remain at 527 nm and 511 nm respectively, but the overall lens transmittance is slightly reduced. In 1989 two additional CPF filters were added to the family of CPF filters, increasing the number to seven. CFP 450 was added as an indoor lens to provide moderate short wavelength filtering with a high total transmittance. It has its visible light cutoff at 450 nm and is especially helpful for reading, watching television, and reducing the glare from fluorescent lighting. Outdoors the CPF 450 darkens to approximately 18% in a brown color. At the other end of the spectrum, the addition of the CPF 550XD provided for more protection and filtering than the original CPF 550. The CPF 550XD has a 99% filter attenuation below 550 nm. This lens is useful in extreme and severe cases of photophobia and has found acceptance with patients who have aniridia and achromatopsia. Table 4-2 lists the characteristics of all the Corning CPF filters.

TABLE 4-2
Filter Characteristics

	CPF 450	CPF 511-S	CPF 511-Dn	CPF 527-S	CPF 527-Dn	CPF 550-S	CPF 550-XD
Visible light cutoff	450nm	511nm	511nm	527nm	527nm	550nm	550nm
Filtering below cutoff*	96%	98%	98%	98%	98%	98%	99%
Transmittance lightened	73%	47%	34%	34%	26%	20%	8%
Transmittance darkened	18%	12%	10%	9%	8%	5%	3%
UV Filtering							
UVB	100%	100%	100%	100%	100%	100%	100%
UVA*	97%	99%	99%	98%	99%	99%	99%

* Percentages shown are minimum. Actual values are typically higher.
Reproduced by permission of Corning Inc.

It is recommended that the clinician have a trial kit of filters to demonstrate to patients. Symptoms and patient reaction after trial will guide the clinician to the correct choice of filter. Caution must be exercised in prescribing the CPF filters to ensure that the filter does not significantly interfere with color discrimination. This is especially important in driving situations. These filters are not indicated for night driving and the CPF 550XD is not indicated for daytime driving because it does not meet the ANSI Z80.3 nonprescription sunglass transmittance standards for daytime driving. Its use in daytime driving calls for a careful professional evaluation based on performance for safe driving. Kits are available in Plano lenses with the filters mounted into frames with side shields, as trial lenses for trial frames or use with Halberg clips, and as clip-ons to fit over existing eyewear.

Younger Protective Lens Series (PLS filters)

Younger Optics developed the Protective Lens Series to provide selective filtering protection from ultraviolet and blue light. These CR-39 filters are designated PLS 530, PLS 540, and PLS 550, and their numerical designation indicates the cutoff point below which almost all ultraviolet and visible light is attenuated. The PLS 530 is an orange-amber filter, the PLS 540 is a brown filter, and the PLS 550 is a reddish-orange filter. Being manufactured in CR-39, the lenses have the advantages of a plastic lens over a glass lens, but also have their disadvantages. One major difference between the PLS series and the CPF series is that the PLS series is not photochromic. Younger indicates that these lenses can be given a cosmetic tint by regular tinting methods and this will not cause any change in the absorptive properties of the lens. Table 4-3 lists the specifications of the PLS series.

NoIR Medical Technologies

NoIR Medical Technologies manufactures a wide variety of filters that are useful for many low vision conditions. These nonprescription filters are made of plastic. Frames are available in both standard and fit-over goggle style. The total visible transmission varies from 1% to

TABLE 4-3
Younger Protective Lens Series (PLS)

Filter	Visible transmittance at 400 nm	Visible transmittance at 700 nm
PLS 530	5%	89%
PLS 540	1%	68%
PLS 550	1%	90%

90%. Table 4-4 lists the filters and the styles in which they are available.

Studies to determine preferences for the 100 series with various low vision pathologies, show the widest acceptance for Model 101,

TABLE 4-4
NoIR Medical Technologies Filters

Color of filter	Total light transmission	Models (see codes below)*						
Dark Grey-Green	1%	108	208	408		708		
Dark Amber	2%	107	207	407	507	707		
Dark Red	4%						U93	
Plum	4%			480			U80	
Dark Amber	4%						U43	
Dark Grey-Green	4%						U33	
Dark Grey	4%						U23	
Dark Orange	4%						U63	
Dark Yellow	4%						U53	
Grey-Green	7%			430			U30	S30
Medium Amber	10%	101	201	401	501	701		
Dark Grey	13%			422			U22	S22
Amber	16%						U40	S40
Medium Green	18%	102	202	402	502	702		
Medium Plum	20%						U81	
Medium Grey	32%			421			U21	S21
Light Plum	40%						U88	
Light Grey Green	40%	112	212		512	712		
Light Amber	40%	111	211	411	511	711		
Pink	44%						U70	
Red	45%			490			U90	
Orange-Red	47%						U75	
Orange	49%			460			U60	S60
Light Grey-Green	50%						U38	
Light Orange	52%						U68	
Light Amber	53%						U48	
Yellow	54%			450			U50	S50
Light Grey	58%						U28	
Light Grey	58%			420			U20	S20
Light Yellow	65%						U58	
Clear	90%		210	410			U10	S10

* Model Codes:
  100 Series > Regular Fit Over
  200 Series > Wrap-around Frame
  400 Series > Fashion Frames, Adult & Pediatric, Clip-ons
  500 Series > Large Fit Overs
  700 Series > Medium Fit Overs
  U- Series > UV Shields—regular
  S- Series > UV Shields—small
Filter Designation: First digit is Model Series, second and third digit indicate filter color/transmission.
For example: "430" indicates a "400 Series" Fashion frame or clip-on in Grey-Green 7% transmission. The U30 and S30 show similar transmission in the UV shield and Small UV Shield.

followed by Model 102 and Model 107. Diabetics seem to prefer Model 101 and Model 102.

Other Forms of Light Control

Besides lights and filters there are many other devices that can be used to reduce glare and control illumination. The typoscope is one of the simplest light control devices (Figure 4-6). Prentice described the original typoscope as a device which "excludes all light reflected from the surface of the paper except that which actually affords the necessary contrast between it and the type within the slot."[11] The typoscope is a very useful light control device and can also be used as a place finder or guide. The addition of a small piece of yellow acetate filter can add additional contrast similar to a Hi-Liter marking pen. The use of the typoscope with a small portable high-intensity lamp is

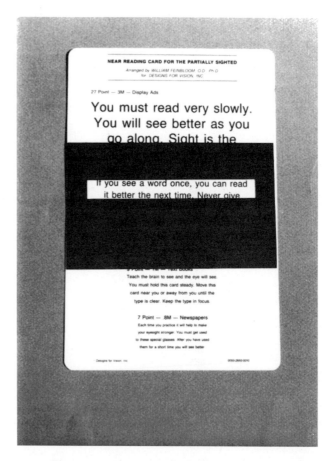

FIGURE 4-6 The typoscope can be used as both a light control device and an aid to help keep one's place while reading. (Photo courtesy of Designs for Vision Inc. Ronkonkoma, NY.)

an excellent way to provide the needed contrast and reduce extraneous glare. The typoscope aids in providing the optimum ratio of ground illumination to detail illumination. Typoscopes can be made out of a variety of material such as black posterboard, black acetate sheets, or black construction paper. The vertical depth of the slot should be large enough to permit two to three lines of print to be seen at one time, and the slot should be wide enough so that horizontal movement of the typoscope is not required. Typoscopes of various sizes can be made for books, newspapers, or magazines depending on the layout of the material. The edges of the slot should be cut clean with a razor blade to prevent ragged edges that could cause distraction.

Multiple pinhole glasses have been found to be effective for patients with irregular corneas or with opacities of the ocular media where the macular function is still intact. The pinhole utilizes the principle of paraxial rays, limiting the size of the retinal blur circle and enhancing contrast definition. Fonda[12] recommends that the size of the pinhole diameter range from .5 to 1.5 mm, with about 1 mm being most effective. Smaller pinholes limit the retinal illumination, and larger pinholes are not effective in creating the paraxial ray effect. The distance between the holes should not be larger than the patient's pupillary diameter to avoid monocular diplopia. The average distance between holes is approximately 3.5 mm. Caution must be exercised in using pinholes with macular pathology because the retinal illumination can be considerably reduced. The disadvantage of this form of light control is that the glasses are somewhat unattractive and for best effect must be worn in bright illumination.

Controlled pupil contact lenses and pinhole contact lenses are described in detail by Rosenbloom.[13] He states that the controlled pupil contact lens acts to pass only the paraxial rays while restricting rays which may be dispersed by the media. The reduction of light by the pupil lens may allow the pupil to dilate, thus allowing vision around an opacity. This form of light control has been useful for patients with aniridia, coloboma of the iris, scarred corneas, diffuse corneal opacities, subluxation of the lens, and for general cosmetic improvement of disfigured eyes.

Stenopaic slits have been used for centuries as a form of light control. Gregg[14] describes goggles, worn by the Eskimos, that were carved out of wood with a narrow slit. Cohen and Waiss[15] reported that horizontally louvered lenses can act as effective glare reducing devices for patients who have medial opacities. Consideration must be given, however, to the loss of visual field and the loss of retinal illumination. This is especially true in situations where the outdoor illumination may suddenly be reduced.

Hats, visors, clip-ons, and umbrellas can act as light control devices. A simple baseball cap with a wide brim will offer overhead glare protection and often improve the performance of a pair of sunglasses used alone. The cap with a wide brim is one device many patients will readily accept because it is not an unusual device and does not draw attention to their visual impairment.

Posture and Positioning Devices

A prescribed low vision device must be comfortable. With many low vision systems, the maintenance of focal distance, line of sight, head tilt, back position, and body posture determine the comfort and efficiency of the prescribed aid. Postural modifications can often be made to improve the performance of low vision devices. The correct posture will often be dictated by the nature of the low vision prescription. Howard and Templeton[16] believe that postural reflexes are concerned with the positions and relationships of various parts of the body. They contend that the eyes, touch receptors in the skin, muscles, tendons, joints, and the vestibular apparatus all contribute to total postural-reflex behavior.

> **CLINICAL PEARL**
>
> *With many low vision systems, the maintenance of focal distance, line of sight, head tilt, back position, and body posture determine comfort and efficiency of the prescribed aid.*

With a few exceptions, most low vision devices require a short or close working distance and/or a modification in head position and line of sight to achieve success. Working distance is defined as the distance between the object of regard and the standard spectacle plane. When relative distance magnification is utilized, there is a decrease in working distance. The higher the power of the aid, the more critical it is to maintain the material at the correct focal distance.

When there are concurrent problems of arthritis, Parkinson's disease, manual dexterity, muscular weakness, or other infirmities, patients may tire when attempting to hold the material at the proper distance. Postural reflexes and muscular input produce feedback which often results in moving the material to a more comfortable position, causing the print to go out of focus. The proper positioning and maintenance of this positioning are essential for success.

Individuals vary in the way they hold books, magazines, or newspapers. There is less distortion when the material is positioned so that the line of sight can be perpendicular to the page. As the reading material is tilted downward and away from the perpendicular, the visual perception becomes increasingly distorted. Tinker[17] has shown that for the reader who sits upright, the normal and comfortable line of sight is perpendicular to the plane of the copy when the material is tilted approximately 45 degrees up from the table top or down from the vertical. As the position varies from 45 degrees, sloping away from the vertical, visibility decreases. Reading stands, racks, lapboards, trays, and easels all provide improved posture and maintenance of position to allow functional use of the prescribed aid.

Ordinary reading stands or book racks (Figure 4-7) may be sufficient for some patients. Merely propping up the book so the patient does not have to bend over will create less back strain. When the depth of focus is not too critical, these book racks may be used.

Occasionally the material needs to be brought close to the eyes in conjunction with other tasks that are occurring simultaneously. Such tasks may include entering data into a computer by typing from copy. While typing can be done at a longer distance, the working distance to the copy may have to be reduced. Flexible and movable stands may prove to be the solution in these cases (Figure 4-8). One disadvantage of this type of stand, however, is that many of them are incapable of holding much weight.

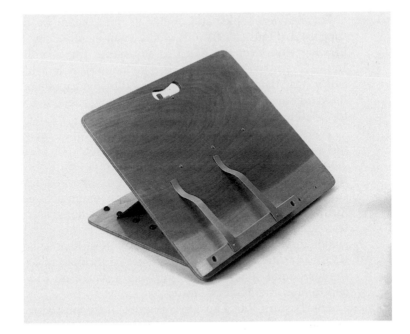

FIGURE 4-7 APH Desktop Reading Stand. This stand provides for a wide working area and is adjustiable to several tilt positions. (Photo reproduced courtesy of American Printing House for the Blind, Inc.)

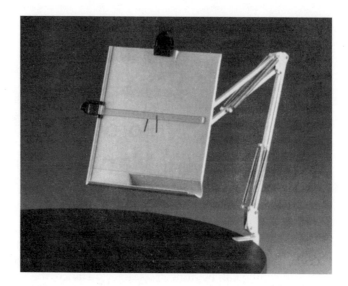

FIGURE 4-8 Luxo Copy Holder. This stand holds copy and is adjustable over a wide range of reading distances. The stand has a line guide for keeping one's place. (Photo courtesy of The Lighthouse Inc.)

For heavier books and material, the Shafer Reading Stand is suggested (Figure 4-9). This stand, manufactured by the American Printing House for the Blind, is adjustable, free-standing, and has a 16″ × 12″ tray with a small shelf. The height is adjustable to 44 inches and it has a lateral movement with extension capability to 27 inches. Its sturdy steel construction and heavy base make it a valuable asset for holding charts during the examination.

When there is a necessity to hold the material upright in front of the patient's eyes, a table easel may be used. The Desktop Reading Stand (Fig. 4-7), also manufactured by American Printing House for the Blind, is a wooden stand capable of five position angles. The surface measures 18″ × 23¾″. Eschenbach manufactures the wooden Reading Desk which has four adjustable positions, an optional accessory guide rail, and a surface size of 40 × 35 cm. Other inexpensive stands include the Easy Reader and the Easi-Reader Bookstand. The K&L EZ Writer is a slanted work surface inclined at 20 degrees from the horizontal. It is made of lightweight plexiglass and comes with a clip to hold the material steady.

The Posture Rite Lap Desk (Figure 4-10) provides an adjustable nonglare, laminated surface which is attached to a fabric cushion. The cushion conforms to the lap and is adjustable from a flat surface to a 20 degree tilt. The top size measures 15½″ × 13¼″.

Reading in bed can present problems for posture and position. The Mydesc Custom Desktop may provide a solution to this particular

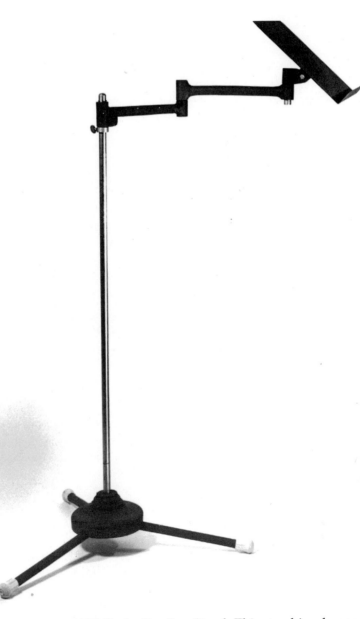

FIGURE 4-9 APH Shafer Reading Stand. This stand is a heavy duty stand capable of holding oversize and other heavy books. It is completely adjustable and comes with a weighted base. (Photo courtesy of American Printing House for the Blind Inc.)

problem. It is an ergonomically designed desktop which consists of a base that fits between the box spring and mattress. It is completely adjustable and capable of tilting to a number of positions. It is also adaptable to wheelchairs.

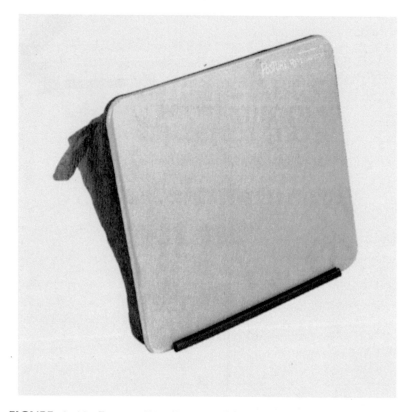

FIGURE 4-10 Posture-Rite Lap Desk. This product is helpful for patients who need a flat working surface. It is also helpful for patients who are bedridden. (Photo courtesy of The Lighthouse Inc.)

Ergonomic design has been incorporated into some of the newer designs of hand magnifiers. Designs for Vision, Inc. has designed some of its Clear Image lenses with an ergonomic handle that allows for comfortable prolonged use (Figure 4-11). COIL has designed some of its new magnifiers with special handles that reduce the fatigue caused by continued use. Additional companies will soon learn that comfort and posture will be factors important beyond just the lens design.

Special ring stands, clamps, and headbands can be used to position monoculars and binoculars prescribed for prolonged use. When critical positioning is needed with a monocular prescribed for near viewing, the device can be positioned in front of the eye with a ring stand. Tripods and stands may be needed for telescopic systems above 8× to allow steady prolonged viewing. Walters provides headbands that can accommodate monoculars or be custom fitted for other telescopic devices (Figure 4-12).

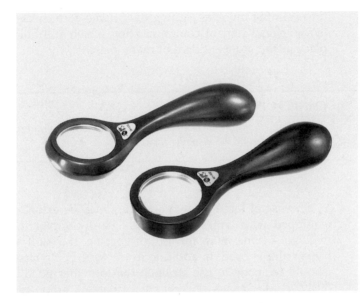

FIGURE 4-11 Designs for Vision Hand Held Clear Image Magnifiers. This product has an ergonomically designed handle to reduce fatigue. (Photo courtesy of Designs for Vision, Inc., Ronkonkoma, NY.)

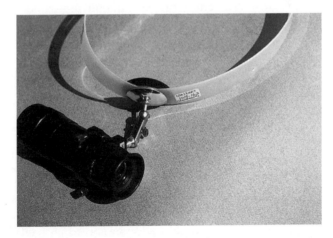

FIGURE 4-12 Head band mounting for telescopic device. The head band with a swivel joint allows freedom in positioning.

Writing and Communication Devices

Adaptation of simple devices used every day for communication has made this task easier for the visually impaired. These patients often complain they cannot handle their own personal affairs, which oftentimes simply involves signing their name on a check. Writing a letter is a personal part of communication which still holds an important place in the independence of many patients.

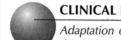

CLINICAL PEARL

Adaptation of simple devices used every day for communication has made this task easier for the visually impaired.

The use of large print typewriters may be extended to computers equipped with large font output. The development of typing skills will go a long way toward preserving the skill of writing. If a typewriter is used, in addition to the type being large, modifications should be made to use a ribbon that provides good contrast. Special heavily inked black ribbons are available. Carbon ribbons are also a good choice. On the computer, a laser printer provides a good clean image. A bold, sans serif font is desirable.

Being able to write and read one's signature is important. Keeping the letters and words on the line while writing and making clearly distinguishable letters can be difficult unless adaptations are made. The use of handwriting guides, signature guides, or stencils can help. The signature guide is very similar to a typoscope and is usually made of plastic with an opening to correspond to the standard signature area. These signature guides can be custom made to fit a particular form, or with the assistance of a sighted person, placed on a blank form in the appropriate position for the signature. These check guides are premade for the standard $3\frac{3}{4}''\times 6''$ check. Other guides can be made for addressing envelopes. Rigid signature guides use two thin aluminum rods approximately $\frac{1}{2}$ inch apart. These guides give stability and security to unsteady hands. The rubber block feet prevent the guide from slipping on the paper. One disadvantage of the rigid guide is the constriction it creates in writing certain letters with ascenders such as *d, b, k,* and *t;* or desenders such as *g* and *y*. The problems of the rigid guides can be solved with either the Easy Writer full page writing guide or the Marks Script Guide. The Easy Writer is a stringed frame that holds a standard sheet of $8\frac{1}{2}$-by-11-inch paper. The strings are flexible enough to allow ascenders and desenders to be written without interference. The Marks Script Guide consists of a clipboard with a notched guide and two thin flexible wires allowing for some "give." This guide is especially useful for those who need to develop long handwriting by keeping their place on the line.

Paper can also be modified to provide contrast and spacing. Besides providing a location on the page and guide for the user, contrast can be provided with bold lined paper. Bold line or heavy line paper is available from the American Printing House for the Blind and many other sources. Types of bold line paper differ in the thickness of the lines and spacing (Figure 4-13). Low vision writing paper is available with very bold thick lines which are $\frac{9}{16}$ inch apart. Thick line paper is available with line separations of $\frac{3}{4}$ inch and $\frac{1}{2}$ inch. Notebook paper is 50 pound standard paper finish with a left hand margin. APH paper is available in four styles: beginner's writing paper, green-lined paper, notebook paper, and letter writing paper. The latter comes with lines either $\frac{2}{16}$ apart or $\frac{9}{16}$ apart. Tactile or raised line writing paper is available for tactile clues. Simply folding the paper to provide creases will occasionally provide a tactile line for guidance.

To be most functional for the visually impaired, pens should have high contrast. Felt tip markers or pens with bold easy-to-read black ink should be considered. Special pens include the 20/20 pen with an extra wide, soft bullet tip and the Nitewriter pen which has a built-in spotlight illuminating the writing area. For patients with manual dexterity problems, arthritis, or paresis, larger body pens or pens inserted into handheld balls may provide enough grip to accomplish the writing task.

Medical Assistive Devises

The concurrent presence of other medical conditions which demand monitoring and control is common within the low vision community. The leading cause of legal blindness is diabetic retinopathy, and the

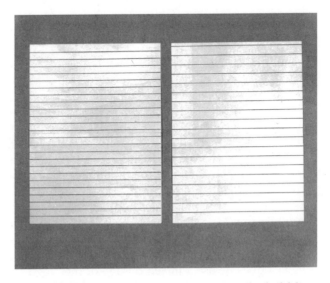

FIGURE 4-13 Letter-writing paper from APH. The bold lines on this 50 pound standard finish paper allow for excellent contrast. (Photo courtesy of American Printing House for the Blind, Inc.)

management and control of diabetes is a major concern for many visually impaired persons. Other tasks involved with medical management and control may consist of timing, matching for color, reading scales, and identification of detail in selecting pills. These tasks all involve visual skills which can be challenging to the visually impaired patient. Taking medications may involve selecting the correct pill or measuring the correct amount of liquid. Filling a syringe with an injection requires being able to correctly see the markings on a scale. Caring for another individual who is ill may involve taking a temperature and reading a thermometer. Monitoring the effectiveness of medications may consist of taking blood pressure and recording the measurements.

CLINICAL PEARL

The concurrent presence of other medical conditions which demand monitoring and control is common within the low vision community.

Diabetic Assistive Devices

By far the largest category under medical assistive devices are products designed for the diabetic patient. The problems facing the visually impaired diabetic are basically twofold: (1) accurately measuring doses of insulin which may be single or mixed doses and (2) monitoring blood sugar levels. The practitioner must have some knowledge of the types of insulin in order to manage the measuring of insulin doses. When insulin was first developed, it was manufactured in the "regular" form. This was a fast acting, short duration insulin much like that secreted by the pancreas. Because of its short duration of action and the need to provide a continuous steady level of blood sugar, injections had to be taken three to four times a day. As research continued into the 1930s, time-release insulins were developed. PZI, NPH, Lente, and other slower acting insulins provided a solution to the need for multiple injections. With the advent of DNA technology, human insulin derivative was introduced. The human insulin product differs from the animal source insulins because its structure is identical to the insulin produced by the pancreas and because of the recombinant DNA technique used in its manufacture. As many patients are changed to the human type of insulin, their physicians may need to change dosages. Therefore the gauges used for dosage may need to be reordered. Today it is not uncommon to have a diabetic use a mixed dosage of the "regular" short acting and longer time-release insulins and vary the dosage depending upon the monitored blood glucose levels. Most patients know their dosage levels and how to determine their insulin needs based on blood glucose levels.

CLINICAL PEARL

By far the largest category under medical assistive devices are products designed for the diabetic patient.

Insulin is contained in a glass vial which has a volume of 10 ml. While the shape of the vials may differ somewhat, the volume capacity is the same. The vial comes capped with a rubber diaphragm stopper which is penetrated in the center by the hypodermic syringe. Although all vials contain the same volume of insulin, the concentrations of the insulin can vary. The concentration is measured in units of insulin contained in each ml of liquid. The concentration commonly used today is the U-100. The U-40 and U-80 lesser concentrations have been phased out and are no longer available.

Dosage for insulin is measured in units. The importance of having the correct syringe for the matching type of insulin cannot be overemphasized. The capacity of a 1 cc syringe with U-100 insulin is 100 units. Likewise, a 1 cc with U-40 insulin contains 40 units. A 20-unit dosage using the U-100 syringe will involve taking up $\frac{1}{5}$ of the volume of the syringe whereas the same dosage on the U-40 syringe involves taking $\frac{1}{2}$ the volume of the syringe. The move to a universal single concentration, U-100, will likely solve many of these potential problems.

Magnifiers that have been specifically designed for syringes are available for use. These magnifiers snap onto the syringe itself or onto the insulin vial and magnify the syringe markings from 2X to 3X. Magni-Guide, manufactured by Becton Dickinson Consumer Products; and Insul-eze, manufactured by Palco Labs, magnify the entire scale and accept both the 1 cc and $\frac{1}{2}$ cc syringes.

The Inject-Aid is a device which can be preset by a sighted individual to assist those with unsteady hands in drawing up a preset and consistent dosage. It also holds the insulin bottle and syringe in one unit. The Holdease holds the vial and syringe. Both of these devices are designed to allow the syringe needle to be centered in the vial cap, avoiding bent and blunted needles. Other funnel-like devices such as the Visual Center Aid can be placed atop the vial to center the needle into the vial cap.

When different amounts of insulin are required, devices capable of mixed dosage may be used. The Click-Count Syringe by Supreme Medical is a 1-cc U-100 glass syringe with a notched plunger that clicks. The clicks can be felt and heard to give auditory and tactile feedback to the user. Each click on the Click-Count is 2 units. Its disadvantage is that the glass syringe needs to have a needle attached and the glass syringe must be boiled between uses to resterilize it. The Count-a-Dose by Jordan Medical Enterprises (Figure 4-14) is now manufactured for use with the Becton-Dickinson Lo-Dose ($\frac{1}{2}$-cc) syringe. The device holds one or two bottles of any brand of insulin and makes a distinctive click with each 1-unit increment. Printed instructions and an audiocassette are included. The Load-Matic by Palco Labs uses a 1-cc syringe and has a thumb lever and click wheel for measurement. The thumb lever measures in 10-unit increments and the click wheel measures in 1-unit increments. After the settings are made, the plunger is pulled to achieve the desired dosage. This device has the advantage of measuring large dosages easily.

New diabetics often have the fear of needles and self-injection. Auto-injectors use glass cartridges which are placed into the penlike devices. The dosages are selected and a button is pressed causing the pen to inject the dialed amount of insulin. The major distributors of insulin in the United States—Eli Lilly and Co., Nordisk-USA, and Squibb-Novo—along with syringe manufacturer Becton Dickinson are working on various types of auto-injector pens. On the market presently are the Autopen, NovolinPen, NovoPen, and the Novolin 70/30 Prefilled. Needleless injectors are also available but are much more expensive and require extensive training and preparation. These needleless injectors deliver insulin subcutaneously into a preselected site and have both auditory and tactile clues to monitor dosage.

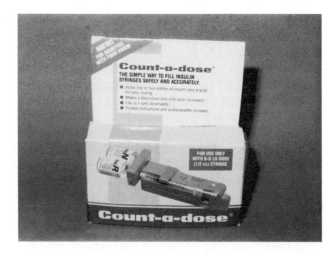

FIGURE 4-14 Count-a-Dose. This diabetic device is designed to hold one or two vials of insulin and provides both tactile and audible clues for proper dosage.

Medijector Tender Touch, Medijector EZ, Preci-jet, Vitajet II, and Freedom Jet are some of the needleless injectors currently on the market.

Devices for monitoring the blood glucose are essential for the visually impaired diabetic. The specific tasks of testing, calibration, control testing, cleaning, and battery replacement need to be emphasized until the procedures become routine. Glucometers equipped with large bold displays, assists for blood placement and amount, and voice output in different languages are now available.

While blood glucose remains the favored method of monitoring in diabetic control, urine testing for glucose is still an appropriate but less reliable option for self-monitoring. Testing for glucose in the urine before each injection, or four times a day at maximum times of insulin action, can help establish patterns and aid in glucose control. For the visually impaired, vision loss can make the required color comparisons in urine testing difficult. Making the color comparison with a white background and additional lighting may prove to be helpful. Large size reagent strips have been discontinued. The Uricator is an electronic device for urine analysis.

Other Medical Assistive Devices

Measuring blood pressure and taking temperatures are two tasks which often present problems for the visually impaired. When there is a concurrent hearing loss, there may be difficulty in hearing the sounds with the use of a stethoscope or reading the gauges on the sphygmomanometer. Jumbo blood pressure meters and thermometers with voice output allow monitoring of temperature and blood pressure. Talking scales and other auditory products will be discussed in the section on sensory adaptive aids, later in this chapter.

Mobility Assistive Devices

Mobility is the basic function of an individual being able to move within the environment. The visually impaired have long relied upon other persons, animals, and implements such as sticks to assist in mobility. Visual acuity should not be the only determinant for mobility assistance. Fonda[18] defines traveling vision as vision of 3/200 or better, if it is assumed that the peripheral field is greater than 50 degrees.

CLINICAL PEARL

Visual acuity should not be the only determinant for mobility assistance.

The constriction of the peripheral field, however, undoubtedly plays a greater role and Faye[19] states that a patient needs 20 degrees or more of central field to allow rapid orientation in familiar surroundings. Today when an individual does not have enough vision to travel with ease, assistance may be provided in basically four different ways. The first and probably the simplest form of assistance is the use of a sighted guide. The second is the use of canes or the long cane of various lengths. The third is the use of dog guides, and the fourth involves the use of electronic mobility devices.

Many blind and severely visually impaired persons get around with the help of others. It is important for the low vision practitioner to know the proper techniques for assisting a blind individual in mobility. When walking with an individual who desires assistance, keep the guiding arm close to the side with the elbow bent. The visually impaired traveler should walk about a half step behind, firmly holding the sighted person's arm just above the elbow. The guide should stay about one step ahead, but avoid being too far ahead as to require the visually impaired individual to "catch up." The bent elbow should be placed behind the back to signal narrow passageways, doors, or crowded areas. The visually impaired person can, with the guide's arm in this position, feel and easily follow movements in a safe manner.

Vocabulary must be carefully phrased when assisting. Avoid phrases like: "over there," "there it is," or "it's right here." Instead, use specific terminology such as: "toward," "away," "directly in front of you," "directly to your right or left," or "behind you." If you leave the visually impaired individual alone, he or she should be put in contact with a chair, a wall, or other object. This makes it possible to become oriented with the enviroment. Keep in mind that conversation with these individuals does not require shouting. While they may be visually impaired, many have normal audition.

Canes

There are several types of canes which are commonly used by the visually impaired. The stereotyped picture of a blind person includes the white cane. In reality, canes can be long canes, folding or collapsible canes, white wooden canes, or support canes. They can be constructed out of wood, aluminum, plastic, fiberglass, graphite, or stainless steel. The cane provides both an extension of tactile kinesthetic sense and a form of protection to the user.

The long cane was developed in the 1940s by Richard Hoover and differs from an orthopedic cane, which was used prior to its introduction. The long cane has no support function, but rather is used to sense the immediate environment and provide clues useful for mobility (Figure 4-15). Canes vary in length, but ideally the length should be sufficient to provide the user with feedback clues about the surroundings in enough time to react, but not limit the user's mobility.

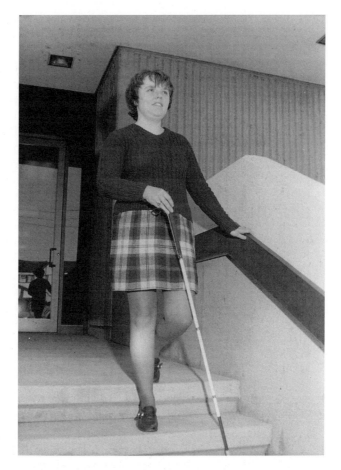

FIGURE 4-15 Mobility Cane. The long cane provides tactile clues to the immediate environment at the point of contact and requires special training to become proficient in its use.

When measuring for a cane, the usual length is taken from the ground at the side of the foot in a forward position to $1\frac{1}{2}$ inch above the bottom of the sternum.

CLINICAL PEARL

The long cane has no support function, but rather is used to sense the immediate environment and provide clues useful for mobility.

The long canes are available in basically two types: nonrigid (folding or telescopic) and rigid. Nonrigid canes consist of sections of metal or fiberglass tubing held together by an inner mechanism such as an elastic cord, knurled friction joints, or a steel tension cable. Rigid canes typically have solid fiberglass or hollow aluminum shafts. Canes can have either straight or crooked handles.

One disadvantage of the long cane is that it does not provide information concerning the environment until the cane makes contact. Since the cane is directed downward, there is no forewarning concerning overhead obstacles and thus no protection is offered to the upper part of the body. The basic technique in cane travel involves the rhythmic movement of the cane in an arc pattern in front of the body. This deceptively simple technique requires extensive training for the full utilization and potential of the cane to be realized. Once the long cane is mastered, its user can walk erect at a normal pace in unfamiliar environments without sight or assistance. When there is partial sight, some patients use white canes (often the orthopedic type) as identification and as a sign to sighted travelers that they have a visual impairment.

Dog Guides

The use of dogs as mobility aids dates back centuries. In the United States, however, it was not until 1929 that the first formal training of blind students to work with dogs for mobility purposes was organized by Dorothy Harrison Eustis.[20]

There are many components of a dog guide program, including selection and breeding of dogs, training of the dogs and instructors, matching dogs and users, mobility team training, and research. The use of a dog guide requires extensive training as well as maturity and intelligence on both the part of the dog and user. Regular exercise and proper care are important for the dogs. Because of this, people who qualify for dogs are usually between the ages of 18 and 60, in good health, with good hearing, and without residual vision which might hinder the use of a dog.

CLINICAL PEARL

The dog guide program includes selection and breeding of dogs, training of the dogs and instructors, matching dogs and users, mobility team training, and research.

Dog guides (*dog guide* is the proper term and is generic; *guide dogs* refer to dog guides from the dog guide school in San Raphael, California) are not for every blind or partially sighted person. Some prefer the dog guides as a means of travel because the dog can protect the person from hazards that might not be detected by a long cane. Many diabetics for this reason prefer a dog to the long cane as a mobility aid. Diabetics must be careful to guard themselves against personal injury.

Because of the rigorous job that the dog guide is called upon to perform, temperament, trainability, and size must be taken into consideration in selection of the dog. In general, the common breeds that are used for dog guides include the German shepherd, the golden retriever, the Labrador retriever, and boxers. Dogs must be easily groomed and this eliminates many longhair breeds. Female dogs are preferred because they seem to have more even and gentle temperaments and are more easily trained.

Electronic Travel Aids (ETAs)

Electronic travel aids (ETAs) provide for additional sensory input for the user and overcome some of the shortcomings of the long cane. In actual use, ETAs probably comprise a very small percentage of the mobility devices used by the low vision and blind populations. The reasons for the nonuse of ETAs are basically threefold: (1) The devices are expensive. Technology, while prominent in the field of sensory devices, has not brought down the cost to where widespread use is common. Less expensive alternatives often substitute and are found to be viable solutions. (2) The additional sensory input provided by many of the ETAs often presents too much sensory information. They may work as a detriment rather than an assist to the user. (3) Additional training and time are required to achieve proficiency with ETAs. These problems lead to a very small pool of users and instructors from whom experience and training (even among certified orientation and mobility instructors) can be gained. Even so, ETAs do offer new alternatives and provide some solutions where other mobility devices seem inappropriate.

CLINICAL PEARL

Electronic travel aids (ETAs) provide for additional sensory input for the user and overcome some of the shortcomings of the long cane.

ETAs for the most part can be grouped into two categories: passive and active. Passive ETAs respond to the ambient light in the environment, whereas active aids radiate a beam or acoustic wave that is sent out into the environment to be reflected back to the receiving portion of the aid. Of the several aids that have been developed, only a small number have survived beyond a prototype stage to actually be used in the field. Three devices that continue to have occasional use are the Pathsounder, the Laser Cane, and the Sonicguide.

The Pathsounder was invented by Lindsay Russell in the 1960s and is an ultrasonic mobility device which has the advantage of detection of obstacles for wheelchair and walker users. The major disadvantage of the Pathsounder is that the device requires extensive training. The device is worn on the chest and positioned by a neck strap. It can be used to provide information on above the waist obstacles when used in conjunction with the long cane. The additional information that the Pathsounder provides is in the form of auditory or vibratory output. An ultrasonic beam is emitted, reflected off an obstacle, detected by the transducers, and converted into a pulsating buzzing sound heard from tiny speakers mounted in the neck strap. An optional vibratory output is available that causes the entire unit to vibrate on the chest and this output changes to the neckstrap when the obstacle comes closer. No output is received when obstacles are out of the detection range (approximately 6 feet) of the device.

The Laser Cane (Nurion), which is occasionally used today (Figure 4-16), grew out the developments of early research with optical triangulation in 1943. Using this principle, objects are detected and their range and height above ground are determined. Many developments and prototypes as well as field testing and miniaturization eventually led to the introduction of the C5 Laser Cane. It is essentially a long cane with built-in secondary detection capabilities for early warning of hazards. The cane is equipped with three small lasers that emit pulses from 40 to 80 times per second. The beam is so highly collimated that it is only 1 inch wide at a 10 foot distance. Because of this feature, obstacles can be detected and located with a high degree of accuracy. The three lasers are positioned into "channels." The upper channel detects obstacles at head height approximately $2\frac{1}{2}$ feet in front of the cane tip; the straight ahead channel is approximately 2 feet above the ground and ranges out to a maximum distance of 5 to 12 feet from the cane tip; and the downward channel is directed approximately 3 feet beyond the tip of the cane or about 6 feet in front of the user to detect any dropoff greater than 5 inches. Interruptions in the beam are detected by photosensors and converted into different pitched auditory tones to warn of impending hazards. The main criticism of the Laser Cane is that the tonal output may interfere with the natural sensory processing provided by the long cane alone. This, along with the expense, has resulted in limited use of the Laser Cane.

The Sonicguide (binaural sensory aid) was developed by Dr. Leslie Kay. It is manufactured by Wormald International in New Zealand. Sonicguide is a trade name for the manufacturer's commercial product. The term *binaural sensory aid* is a generic name for a group of aids using a similar concept with varying uses and designs. The Sonicguide grew out of the early developments of an ultrasonic, one-channel output device called the Sonic Torch. Modifications of the Sonic Torch to add another output channel and mount the device into

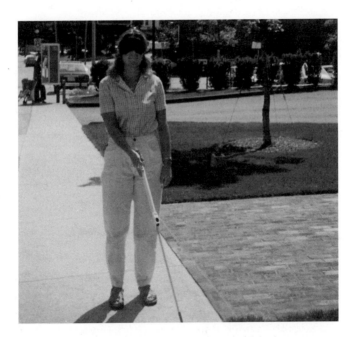

FIGURE 4-16 Laser Cane in use. Three invisible beams are emitted from the laser cane: an upper beam, a straight ahead beam, and a downward beam. There are three distinctly different audible tones which correspond to the light beams when an object is encountered. (Photo reproduced with permission of Sally Jo Sager, MA.)

spectacles created the binaural sensory aid (BSA), which has come to be known as the Sonicguide.

The device has a small transducer located in the eyeglass frame which transmits ultrasonic beams. When beams are reflected off an obstacle, they are received by the microphones and converted into audible sounds conducted by ear tubes so as not to obstruct normal hearing. The characteristics of the sound provide information about the distance and surface quality of the obstacle. Although Kay[21] admits the device cannot be used alone as a mobility device, when used with the long cane considerable improvement has been demonstrated. Confusion with false signals continues to be a problem in the use of the Sonicguide with children.

Two other electronic mobility assistive devices include the Mowat Sensor and light probes. The Mowat Sensor, first conceived by Geoffrey Mowat in 1970, is a device which transmits a beam of high frequency ultrasonic waves into the environmental surround. Objects and obstacles in the beam's path are detected and reflected back, causing the Sensor to vibrate silently. The rate and strength of the vibration relate to the size and distance of the object or obstacle. Currently the Mowat Sensor is used as a teaching tool for concept development and as an accessory mobility aid. Light probes are devices containing photoelectric cells that detect light and convert this light energy into other forms of output information via transducers. The usual output sensory channels are either vibratory or auditory.

Illumination and Mobility

Special problems in mobility arise in retinitis pigmentosa (RP). In advanced cases of RP, with reduced illumination, the patient is forced to use a reduced peripheral field, a small central field, and a nonfunctional scotopic sensitivity. Many RP patients report "night blindness" under dim photopic conditions. This is supported by the fact that many of these patients show high cone thresholds and abnormal cone function in the early stages of the progressive degeneration. These patients often are very light sensitive and need high photopic conditions for optimum mobility. Three devices have shown potential for assisting the RP patient.

The Wide Angle Mobility Light (WAML), manufactured by Innovational Rehabilitation Technology, is a wide angle flashlight worn at waist level to illuminate the path and provide lighting to enhance mobility under dim illumination (Figure 4-17). Morrisette et al.[22] reported that the WAML reduced the rate of error in helping night

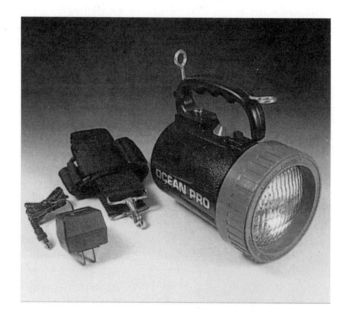

FIGURE 4-17 Wide Angle Mobility Light (WAML). This mobility light provides approximately 1400 candlepower and has a rechargeable battery to enhance night mobility. (Photo courtesy of The Lighthouse Inc.)

blind subjects when tested in a mobility course of residential streets at night.

Nightscope technology grew out of some of the early technology and research done at the U.S. Army Night Vision Laboratory (having a history back to the "sniperscope" of World War II). Today nightscopes or Night Vision Aids (NVAs) are much more compact and are usually monocular. They have 1X magnification, a focusing range of approximately 40 cm to infinity, and fields of around 40 degrees. NVAs use the technology of both the United States and Russian war efforts. Berson[23] indicates the best subjects for nightscopes are candidates having at least 10 degrees of central field. Patients with fields less than 10 degrees may not demonstrate improved mobility with NVAs. Although the size and weight of the NVA is an advantage over the WAML, a significant disadvantage is the cost. The Moonwalker is a compactly-sized new product which is currently in production. It weighs only 12 ounces (Figure 4-18). The field of view on the Moonwalker is approximately 20 degrees, amplifies 1000 times, and has an eyepiece adjustment of +/− 4.00 D. The cost of the Moonwalker is also significantly less than comparable larger NVAs.

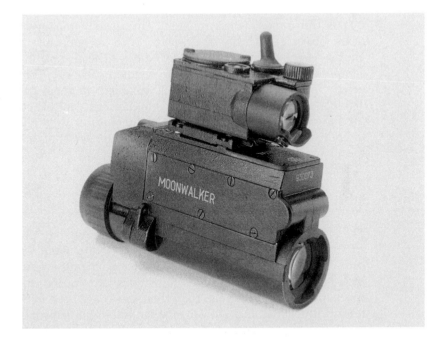

FIGURE 4-18 Moonwalker. This is a palm-sized night scope which amplifies light approximately 1000 times and easily fits into a pocket or purse. (Photo courtesy of Moonlight Products, Inc., San Diego, Calif.)

CLINICAL PEARL

Patients with fields less than 10 degrees may not demonstrate improved mobility with night visual aids (NVAs).

Other high-intensity and wide angle lights have been used for improving mobility. The distribution of the light pattern, the brightness, and several other factors must be taken into consideration in selecting a night mobility device. In a study by Robinson,[24] it was indicated that no one night light is best for all individuals and in some cases, a high-intensity light may be preferable to a wide angle light.

Functional assistance for visually impaired and blind persons in mobility and orientation will advance with future technology. Currently being developed are devices that utilize military global satellites to determine an individual's exact location.[25] These "personal navigation systems" will call out the location of objects as an individual navigates through an environment. The signals from the Global-Positioning System satellites are relayed to an antenna and coordinated with a computerized geographic information system map of the immediate environment. The visually impaired individual hears obstacles identify themselves with recognizable sounds or words. An electronic compass indicates head position, so the computer knows which sounds to send to each ear. Computerized geographic mapping is now being installed on some automobiles. These systems along with other computerized controls could allow for individualized transportation in the future, thus allowing for unlimited mobility for individuals who have been shut out from this form of transportation.

Sensory Substitution Assistive and Adaptive Devices

The majority of the total sensory input is predominantly visual, and is so strong that occasionally other senses modify their responses in accordance with the visual input. However, when the visual sensory input channel is so severely impaired that sensory input is not functional to an individual, the other senses are used in an effort to remain functional. In a similar manner, the improvement of function for the low vision patient often involves the use of sensory substitution devices. These devices and sensory clues other than vision are used every day. Auditory examples are the radio, recordings, spoken conversation, and the sound of television. Olfactory sensory input may be the smell of cooking or burning food, the aroma of perfume, or the smell of a pine tree. Sour milk is a good example of how the sense of taste is a valuable sensory input. The firmness of a handshake, the texture of a piece of cloth, the smoothness of a person's face, or the feeling of the raised dots of braille all involve the sense of touch.

CLINICAL PEARL

The majority of the total sensory input is predominantly visual, and is so strong that occasionally other senses modify their responses in accordance with the visual input.

As to which is the best sensory input substitution for vision, controversy still exists. The two primary senses that are used in visual sensory substitution are tactile substitution and auditory substitution. The choice is largely personal depending upon the experience of the individual and the amount of time and training the patient has brought to the task. Some tests have shown, however, that auditory substitution in the form of synthesized speech can be assimilated more rapidly than other machine outputs—specifically, tactile or nonspeech auditory outputs (beepers or tones).

CLINICAL PEARL

The two primary senses that are used in visual sensory substitution are tactile substitution and auditory substitution.

Auditory Substitution

Next to vision, audition provides the largest sensory input. There are a host of products and services using this sensory form. Examples of auditory substitution for vision include talking books, reader services, audio descriptive services, and a large variety of talking products that use voice output.

CLINICAL PEARL

Examples of auditory substitution for vision include talking books, reader services, audio descriptive services, and a large variety of talking products that use voice output.

Talking books

Talking books are available from many sources as recordings on discs (records), cassettes, and reel-to-reel tape. A major source is the National Library Service for the Blind and Physically Handicapped (NLS). Under the Pratt-Smoot Act, an annual congressional appropriation is made for the provision of talking books and material in other "special media" including large print and braille. Under this act, and along with the passage of Public Laws 89-522 and 89-511, the services for the blind were extended to all persons who are unable to read conventional printed material because of physical and/or visual limitations. This is important, because an individual does not need to be legally blind to qualify for these services. Through NLS, the talking books and other special media material are loaned through a network of national, state, and local libraries.

Most of the talking books available from NLS and other sources are on cassettes. Discs or records and the reel-to-reel have been largely replaced by cassettes. Several magazines are routinely recorded on cassette, including *Fortune, Science, Business Week, Gourmet, Playboy, Popular Science, Popular Mechanics*, the *Smithsonian*, and *Woman's Day*. The NLS publishes a reference circular on *Magazines in Special Media* which lists many sources for recordings. In addition, *Bibles and Other Scriptures in Special Media* and *Volunteers Who Produce Books: Braille-Large Type and Tape*, both from NLS, list numerous sources of recordings. Commercial distribution from such publishers as Thorndike Press/G.K. Hall is available with an extensive collection including current best-selling books.

Standard cassette playback machines may be unsuitable for cassette talking books. Because of the slow speed at which the records are made, playback on special machines may be required to avoid a "Donald Duck" quality. Special machines are available for speeding up the playback without loss of tonal quality. With these speech compressors, the normal conversation rate can be exceeded and approach faster reading rates.

Voice output products

Auditory output is a common feature on many products today. Talking alarm clocks, blood pressure monitors, thermometers, calculators, scales, dictionaries, watches, and glucometers are just a few of the products which may be combined with relative size, color, or illumination to function on more than one sensory level (Figure 4-19). The Voxcom is an audio labeling device that can be used instead of braille or conventional labeling methods. The device consists of a special card, approximately 10 inches in width, that contains magnetic tape upon which a description identification is placed. The cards are attached to an object. When identification is desired, the card is placed into the Voxcom reader which provides for the auditory message of

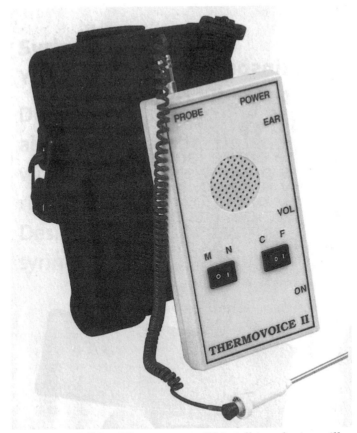

FIGURE 4-19 Talking Thermometer. This talking device will provide an auditory voice output for taking temperature. (Photo courtesy of The Lighthouse Inc.)

identification. The device has a slow reading rate, and approximately 13 words can be placed on the Voxcom card.

Devices that read printed material by optical character recognition are now available. The first such device was an in-line speech adaptor, the Kurzweil Reading Machine. Today Xerox manufactures the Reading Edge, and Arkenstone manufactures the Open Book. Both products have the capacity to scan printed information and read it back or transmit it to computers. Voice outputs can be in one of several languages.

Voice activated phones, the "Note Teller," and computerized speech synthesis demonstrate the sophistication of auditory output. Voice activated phones have the capacity to automatically dial a phone with a voice command. The "Note Teller" identifies U.S. currency from $1 to $100 in clear synthetic speech available in English or Spanish. Voice output modules can convert text normally appearing on a computer screen into speech. These voice output modules have unlimited vocabulary and can vocalize text either as words or letter by letter when typed or displayed. Other products include software that enables the user to have voice output for common commands. The software can be used in conjunction with voice output modules to allow the computer user to have flexible review and command control of the particular programs running on the computer.

More sophisticated yet are the in-line speech adaptors that connect to computers. These devices have not only the ability to vocalize words and letters as they are typed or displayed, but also possess several review features such as identification of cursor position and vocalization of punctuation marks, symbols, strings of numbers, and corrections. Additional product advancements include speech systems in voice output terminals and microcomputers with voice output. A detailed analysis of the particular job functions and needs of the individual is essential in the determination of which technology is used. Output can be in the form of a video screen display, regular print, large print, braille, or synthetic speech.

Other audio assistive products and services

Other audio substitution assistive devices and services include radio/TV services and audio description services. Radio reading services enable the visually impaired to receive information from newspapers, the stock market, weather reports, magazines, and books. Special radio receivers are available for this purpose. Subcarrier closed circuit programs are broadcast and with the use of a special receiver, the information can be heard. The special receiver is necessary because under the current FCC regulations and copyright laws, reading such material over the airwaves is illegal. Radios are now also available that will pick up the audio portion of television broadcasts. This is an excellent method of providing TV auditory information in an inexpensive and portable manner.

Audio Description Service, described by Rockwell and Boris,[26] is a system of low-powered radio equipment that delivers descriptive commentary for theatrical productions. The service is capable of enabling listeners to enjoy live productions at home through the use of FM simulcasts.

Descriptive Video Service (DVS) carefully describes the visual elements of a movie—the action, characters, locations, costumes, and sets. This is done without interfering with the movie's dialogue or sound effects. DVS makes television broadcasts and movies on video available to the blind and visually impaired. DVS is broadcast free to viewers by more than 80 public television stations nationwide. To receive DVS on television, a user must have a stereo TV or VCR that includes the Second Audio Program (SAP) feature or an SAP receiver. When recommending this service to patients, it is advisable to tell them that their VCR should have the capacity not only to receive SAP audio, but also record in the SAP format.

Tactile Substitution

The best example of tactile substitution for vision is braille. Many devices have been developed and marketed utilizing a braille output. Reading machines have been developed with auditory as well as braille outputs. Besides braille, other tactile sensory substitution systems include various paperless braille outputs, and the tactile displays offered in nonbraille format.

CLINICAL PEARL

The best example of tactile substitution for vision is braille; however, other tactile sensory substitution systems include various paperless braille outputs, and the tactile displays offered in nonbraille format.

Braille is a system of printing and writing consisting of haptically distinguishable raised dots that represent letters or symbols of a language.[27] The system of braille, which has been almost universally adopted by blind individuals, was invented by Louis Braille in 1834. Braille is produced in three "grades." Grade I braille consists of material transcribed letter for letter and includes numbers and punctuation marks. It is the simplest grade. Grade II contains all 63 combinations of the basic dot braille cell and contractions and abbreviated words. Grade III braille contains further contracted forms and is used for personal note taking. All three grades utilize the braille cell which contains 6 dot locations in an array 3 high and 2 wide. Depending on the position of the dot in the array, the pattern represents a letter, character, abbreviated word, or contraction.

Most adults will find difficulty in learning braille. In the United States most braille tactile readers are those with severe congenital visual loss who were taught early in life. Congenital blindness favors learning braille more than an adventitious loss. Although some people learn to read braille visually, it is more difficult to become proficient through tactile learning.

Braille readers are doing well if a rate of 100 words per minute is reached. In contrast, talking books approach a conversational rate of around 175 words per minute. Just as in reading printed material, learning to read braille tactilely takes practice and intelligence. With an alert mind and a positive attitude toward learning, reading braille is an achievable goal for some. However, to involve an elderly patient with impaired tactile sensitivity in the task of reading braille for the first time, while commendable, has proven to be less than practical.

Loss of tactile sensitivity is especially important in diabetic patients who may show peripheral neuropathy, creating a loss of touch sensation.

Sources of braille include the National Library Service for the Blind and Physically Handicapped (NLS) and the American Printing House for the Blind (APH). Problems with braille include lack of availability or waiting for a particular selection to be transcribed from a volunteer group if not immediately available from either NLS or APH.

Paperless braille

Braille that is produced without actual impression upon paper is termed *paperless braille*. Instead of having the braille dots embossed upon paper to be tactilely felt, small pins or rods that can be similarly felt are positioned in the same arrangement as a braille cell. By controlling the position of the pins (e.g., whether a pin is extended or retracted) the various symbols or letters can be reproduced. The positioning of the pin locations can be recorded on magnetic tape. By placing a number of these braille cells in a row, the user can scan up to 30 cells at a time so that braille reading can be accomplished.

Paperless braille displays are common today with devices combining the technology of speech synthesizers and microcomputers with interface computer technology to offer a wide variety of products allowing for many applications. By carefully selecting the features that are important to a particular task, sensory outputs can be provided in braille and this output can also be stored in the computer to be later produced in the form of Grade I or Grade II braille, paperless braille, hard copy regular print, large print, or auditory. With the braille display, blind users have access to desktop computers. Telecommunication devices are also available to allow deaf-blind individuals to have communication access. Optical character recognition available with scanners can produce output in braille, either in a hard copy or paperless form. Software is available whereby a braille embosser can produce graphics. Other devices allow direct braille character translation into regular print format.

Nonbraille tactile output

Nonbraille tactile output is used in the Optacon II. The Optacon II (*OP*tical-to-*TA*ctile *CON*verter) is an optical device that converts the information input to a tactile output display (Figure 4-20). The machine has a small miniature camera that is moved across a line of print. The index finger of the user's other hand is placed on a tactile array, which is approximately $\frac{1}{2}$ inch wide and 1 inch long. As the camera is moved across a line of print, the image is reproduced on the tactile array of 100 miniature vibrating rod-stimulator pins. These pins are arranged in rows and columns. The camera consists of 100 light sensitive phototransistors. There is a one-to-one correspondence and

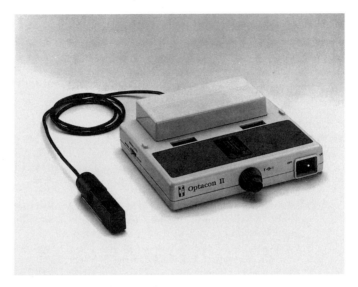

FIGURE 4-20 Optacon II. This sensory substitution product converts optically perceived characters into a tactile array in the form of 100 vibrating sensor pins which are felt by the user. (Photo courtesy of TeleSensory, Mountain View, Calif.)

the reader feels whatever image is viewed by the camera lens. Controls include a zoom lens adjustment and a stimulator intensity control that adjusts the strength of the vibrations. Computer output can be directed into the Optacon for a tactile output. A 3-button mouse is used to scan the material on a PC screen.

Reading speeds with the Optacon II are slow.[28] In one study the average reading speed ranged from 30 to 60 words per minute. Despite this drawback, Optacon II is still one of the most widely used sensory substitution devices. It gains its popularity in allowing the visually impaired to read correspondence, memoranda, notes, and brief messages on an occupational and personal level. It allows privacy. In addition, the device is portable and allows access to material which might be difficult or impossible to transcribe into braille.

Vision Substitution Systems

In recent years scientists and bioengineers have been working toward vision substitution systems. These systems receive visual information which is then converted electronically to another sensory modality which in turn transmits the information directly into the visual cortex. The search for a "neural prosthesis" is still a few decades away. Obstacles to its development include dealing with the presence of a foreign object in the body, the need for a fuller understanding of how the process of vision takes place in the brain, and patient acceptance. Past research of Bach-Y-Rita et al,[29] Brindley,[30] Dobelle,[31-32] and Donaldson,[33] and the present field of bioengineering and robotics will undoubtedly lead to the development of a commercially available neural prosthesis vision substitution system; but for now, most of these devices are products for the future rather than the present.

References

1. Prince J: *Typography for the low vision reader*, Cleveland, 1965, Penton Publishing Co.
2. Fonda G: *Management of the patient with subnormal vision*, St Louis, 1965, Mosby, 6-10.
3. Johnston AW: Making sense of the M, N, and logMAR systems of specifying visual acuity. In Rosenthal BP, Cole RG (eds): *Problems in optometry*, Philadelphia, 1991, Lippincott, 401.
4. Borish IM: *Clinical refraction*, ed 2, Chicago, 1954, Professional Press, 455.
5. Gorn RA, Kuwabara T: Retinal damage by visible light: a physiologic study, *Arch Ophthalmol* 77:115-118, 1967.
6. Kuwabara T, Gorn RA: Retinal damage by visible light: an electron microscopic study, *Arch Ophthalmol* 79:69-78, 1968.
7. Noell WK: Aspects of experimental and hereditary retinal degeneration. In Graymnore CN (ed): *International symposium on the biochemistry of the retina*, London, 1965, Academic Press, 51-72.
8. Dowling JE, Sidman RL: Inherited retinal dystrophy in the rat, *J Cell Biol* 14:73-109, 1962.
9. Berson EL: Light deprivation for early retinitis pigmentosa: a hypothesis, *Arch Ophthalmol* 85:521-529, 1971.
10. Adrian W, Everson RW, Schmidt I: Protection against photic damage in retinitis pigmentosa. In Landers MB, Wolbarsht ML, Dowling JE, Laties AM (eds): Retinitis pigmentosa: clinical implications of current research, *Advances in Experimental Medicine and Biology*, vol 77, New York, 1977, Plenum Press, 233-247.
11. Mehr EB: The typoscope by Charles F. Prentice, *Am J Optom Arch Am Acad Optom* 46:885-887, 1969.
12. Fonda G: *Management of the patient with subnormal vision*, St Louis, 1965, Mosby, 74.
13. Rosenbloom AA: The controlled-pupil contact lens in low vision problems, *J Am Optom Assoc* 40:836-840, 1969.
14. Gregg JR: *The story of optometry*, New York, 1965, Ronald Press, 54.
15. Cohen JM, Waiss B: An evaluation of horizontally louvered black sunwear for glare reduction in a glare sensitive low vision population, *J Vis Rehab* 5(2):61-68, 1991.
16. Howard IP, Templeton WR: *Human spatial orientation*, New York, 1966, Wiley.
17. Tinker MA: Effect of sloped text upon the readability of print, *Am J Optom Arch Am Acad Optom* 33:189-195, 1956.
18. Fonda G: *Management of the patient with subnormal vision*, St Louis, 1965, Mosby, 3.
19. Faye EE: *Clinical low vision*, Boston, 1976, Little, Brown & Co, 243.
20. Whitstock R: Dog guides. In Welsh RL, Blasch BB (eds): *Foundations of orientation and mobility*, New York, 1980, American Foundation for the Blind, 565-580.
21. Kay L: The sonic glasses evaluated, *New Outlook for the Blind* 67:7-11, 1973.
22. Morrisette DL, Goodrich, GL, Marmor MF: A study of the effectiveness of the wide angle mobility light, *J Vis Impairment Blindness* 79:109-111, 1985.
23. Berson EL, Rabin AR, Mehaffey L: Advances in night vision technology: a pocket-scope for patients with retinitis pigmentosa, *Arch Ophthalmol* 90:427-431, 1973.
24. Robinson J, Story SM, Kuyk T: Evaluation of two night-vision devices, *J Vis Impairment Blindness* 84:539-541, 1990.

25. Golean D: Leading the blind. In Focus on Science, *Orange County Register,* September 14, 1994.
26. Rockwell MW, Boris A: Theater and television come to life through audio description, *J Vis Impairment Blindness* 76:320-322, 1982.
27. Goldish LH: *Braille in the United States: its production, distribution, and use,* New York, 1976, American Foundation for the Blind.
28. Goldish LH, Taylor HE: The Optacon: a valuable device for blind persons, *New Outlook for the Blind* 68:49-56, 1974.
29. Bach-y-Rita P, Collins CC, White B, et al: A tactile vision substitution system, *Am J Optom Arch Am Acad of Optom* 46:109-111, 1969.
30. Brindley GS: Effects of electrical stimulation of the visual cortex, *Human Neurobiology* 1:281-283, 1982.
31. Dobelle WH: Current status of research on providing sight to the blind by electrical stimulation of the brain, *J Vis Impairment Blindness* 71:290-297, 1977.
32. Dobelle WH, Mladejovsky MC: The directions of future research on sensory prosthesis, *Transactions of the American Society for Artificial Internal Organs* 20B:425-429, 1974.
33. Donaldson PEK: Experimental visual prosthesis, *IEE Proc* 120:281-297, 1973.

5

Pharmaceutical Effects on the Management of the Low Vision Patient

Gary E. Oliver

Key Terms

low vision	visual acuity	perceived
medications	pupils	brightness
functional vision	visual field	contrast

Many medications can have adverse effects on the functional vision of the low vision patient. These may be localized ocular or more general systemic consequences which affect visual performance with optical or nonoptical devices utilized in the patient's visual rehabilitation. The adverse effects can impact initial management decisions or, possibly more importantly, alter how well a patient performs with a previously prescribed device after using a new medication. This chapter will summarize the more significant pharmaceutical related reactions of commonly prescribed topical ocular medications and selected systemic medications on the functional vision of the low vision patient. Clinical pearls will highlight the effects these medications may have upon the management of the visual rehabilitation

123

ℬ Braille Institute Library Services

of the low vision patient. This chapter is not intended to be an exhaustive review of pharmacology, and the reader is referred to the more comprehensive references listed at the end of the chapter.

Topical Ocular Medications—General Principles

Any topical medication potentially can affect a patient's functional visual acuity or performance with an optical device for a variety of reasons. These include how the drug's pH, tonicity, vehicle, preservative, dosage frequency, usage chronicity, viscosity, and factors specific to the drug's active chemical compound affect the tear film and corneal epithelium. Other factors include the patient's corneal sensitivity and tolerance for acidity, salinity, etc. These adverse effects may be transient or chronic in nature.

CLINICAL PEARL

Low vision evaluations generally should be performed prior to instilling any medications into the patient's eyes in order to eliminate the risk of adverse reactions which may affect the patient's visual performance.

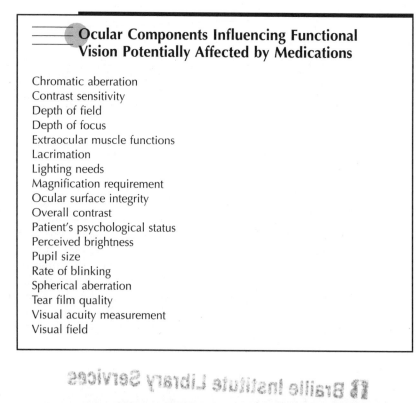

Ocular Components Influencing Functional Vision Potentially Affected by Medications

Chromatic aberration
Contrast sensitivity
Depth of field
Depth of focus
Extraocular muscle functions
Lacrimation
Lighting needs
Magnification requirement
Ocular surface integrity
Overall contrast
Patient's psychological status
Perceived brightness
Pupil size
Rate of blinking
Spherical aberration
Tear film quality
Visual acuity measurement
Visual field

Braille Institute Library Services

> **CLINICAL PEARL**
>
> *Any ophthalmic ointment or solution containing a greater concentration of methylcellulose may temporarily decrease contrast sensitivity and reduce visual acuity.*

> **CLINICAL PEARL**
>
> *Residual effects from ophthalmic ointments may inhibit the patient's ability to successfully wear contact lenses as part of the visual rehabilitation program.*

Anesthetics

Topical anesthetics are used to reduce corneal sensitivity and the patient's blink reflex prior to tonometry or other ocular procedures, such as gonioscopy or corneal foreign body removal. The most commonly used topical anesthetics are proparacaine, benoxinate, and tetracaine. Since these drugs are primarily used for diagnostic purposes, they usually have little effect on the management of the low vision patient.

The adverse ocular effects include transient stinging or burning upon instillation, conjunctival hyperemia, corneal epitheliopathy or sloughing, hypersensitivity reactions to the drug or preservative, and superficial punctate keratitis.

> **CLINICAL PEARL**
>
> *Evaluations performed following instillation of a topical anesthetic may lead to unreliable results due to residual corneal epitheliopathy.*

Mydriatic Agents

Mydriatic drugs are adrenergic agonists which dilate the pupil and facilitate diagnostic evaluation of the lens, retina, choroid, and vitreous. These agents may be direct or indirect acting and produce mydriasis without cycloplegia. Direct acting agents directly stimulate the iris dilator muscle to produce mydriasis, in contrast to indirect acting agents which enhance the release of norepinephrine from the postganglionic neurons. The most commonly used drugs are phenylephrine, which is a direct acting adrenergic agonist, and hydroxyamphetamine, which is an indirect acting agent. Occasionally, phenylephrine is used to help prevent posterior synechiae when treating anterior uveitis. Hydroxyamphetamine is typically used for routine pupillary dilation or the pharmacological workup of anisocoria in Horner's syndrome.

Potential adverse ocular effects include transient stinging upon instillation, blurred vision, photophobia, and hypersensitivity reactions. Systemically, hypertension, myocardial infarction, tachycardia, or other cardiac arrhythmias may occur with 10% phenylephrine. Systemic reactions are uncommon with 2.5% phenylephrine or hydroxyamphetamine.

> **CLINICAL PEARL**
>
> *Visual field testing of glaucoma patients being treated with pilocarpine can be enhanced by instilling phenylephrine or hydroxyamphetamine prior to the procedure. This will usually dilate the miotic pupil from approximately 2 to 4 mm, thereby permitting more accurate visual field analysis.*

Artificial Tears/Ocular Lubricants

Artificial tear and ocular lubricant agents are formulated with either methylcellulose or polyvinyl alcohol related derivatives. These agents are used to manage dry eye syndrome, keratoconjunctivitis sicca, and ocular surface disease. The preparations may be formulated with or without preservatives, isotonic or hypotonic, or electrolyte balanced or nutrient enriched. Preparations containing vitamin A may be beneficial in patients with evidence of squamous metaplasia. Due to the chronic nature of most therapy, nonpreserved agents are preferred when dosage frequency exceeds 4 times per day or when an ointment is prescribed.

Adverse ocular effects may include burning or stinging upon instillation depending on solution pH, tonicity, viscosity, or preservative content. Corneal epitheliopathy may occur secondary to chronic preservative exposure.

> **CLINICAL PEARL**
>
> *Quality of vision frequently improves, which may include increased contrast sensitivity or visual acuity, following pharmacological stabilization of the tear film. However, more viscous artificial tear or ocular lubricant formulations may cause a transient reduction in contrast sensitivity or visual acuity.*

Antihistamine/Decongestant Agents

These drugs are generally used to relieve the signs and symptoms of seasonal allergic or mild vernal conjunctivitis, such as itching, redness, conjunctival congestion, or tearing. Decongestant agents may also be useful for symptomatic relief of mild viral conjunctivitis. Topical antihistamines are H_1-antagonists which relieve symptoms by blocking the H_1-receptor site in order to counteract the effects of histamine. Topical antihistamines include antazoline, pheniramine maleate, and levocabastine. Decongestants, such as naphazoline and phenylephrine, are adrenergic agonists (sympathomimetic) compounds which constrict the conjunctival blood vessels, whiten the eye, and reduce the amount of chemical mediators released from the conjunctival capillaries into the tear film.

Adverse ocular effects from topical antihistamines include burning, lacrimation, redness, superficial punctate keratitis, corneal epitheliopathy, and blurred vision. Vasoconstrictor agents have similar effects and also may cause pupillary mydriasis, which is variable depending upon the drug concentration and absorption through the cornea.

CLINICAL PEARL

Superficial punctate keratitis or other ocular surface abnormalities from topical medications may cause decreased contrast sensitivity, hazy vision, and photophobia.

Nonsteroidal Anti-Inflammatory Drugs (NSAIDs) and Mast Cell Stabilizer Agents

NSAIDs and mast cell stabilizing drugs are prescribed to reduce the signs and symptoms of ocular allergy conditions, maintain pupillary dilation during cataract surgery, reduce ocular inflammation, or reduce corneal sensitivity following refractive surgery and other anterior segment procedures. NSAIDs and mast cell stabilizers may also be useful as adjunct therapy when managing dry eye syndrome patients to reduce the levels of immunological chemical mediators in the tear film in cases where the dry eye is associated with ocular allergy. Depending on the particular drug, these agents reduce clinical signs and symptoms either through inhibition of prostaglandin synthesis by blocking the enzyme cyclo-oxygenase or prevention of mast cell degranulation.

Potential adverse ocular effects include burning or stinging upon instillation, lacrimation, superficial punctate keratitis or corneal epitheliopathy, reduced corneal sensitivity, and blurred vision.

CLINICAL PEARL

Quality of vision often improves, which may include increased contrast sensitivity or visual acuity, following appropriate treatment of ocular allergies due to a reduction in the levels of immunological chemical mediators in the tear film which can cause corneal epitheliopathy.

> **CLINICAL PEARL**
>
> *Some dry eye syndrome patients have concurrent low grade allergic reactions which may respond to treatment with NSAIDs or mast cell stabilizers, resulting in a general improvement in quality of vision.*

Antiinfective Agents

Antibiotic, antiviral, and antifungal drugs are prescribed to prevent or treat infections of the eye and adnexa. Antibiotics are used to treat bacterial blepharitis, conjunctivitis, keratitis, dacryocystitis, and other related dermatitis. Antibiotics also are used as prophylactic therapy to prevent infection following ocular trauma. Antiviral agents are usually prescribed to treat *Herpes simplex* infections. Ocular fungal infections are relatively uncommon.

Treatment with these drugs is usually of short duration with only transient adverse ocular reactions. However, in cases where higher concentrations, more frequent dosages, or ointment formulations are needed, the toxic effects are often more severe either due to the specific drug compound or the preservative. This is particularly true for the aminoglycoside agents or if the compound contains benzalkonium chloride. The antiviral and antifungal agents are also exceptionally toxic to the corneal epithelium.

Typical adverse ocular effects include burning or stinging upon instillation, dry eye syndrome, conjunctival hyperemia, hypersensitivity reactions, corneal epitheliopathy, and superficial punctate keratitis.

> **CLINICAL PEARL**
>
> *Toxic epitheliopathy and superficial punctate keratitis related to antiinfective agents are frequently dose related clinical entities. Sensitivity to medication preservatives also can cause these clinical findings.*

Cycloplegic Mydriatic Agents

Cycloplegic drugs are anticholinergic medications prescribed to inhibit accommodation for cycloplegic refractions or treatment of iritis or uveitis. These agents paralyze or inhibit normal functioning of the ciliary and iris sphincter muscles, resulting in loss of accommodation for near point tasks and dilation of the pupil. The weaker drugs, such as tropicamide, are used for routine pupillary dilation during ophthalmoscopy. Cyclopentolate is typically used for cycloplegic refractions. When used to treat uveitis, the stronger drugs—homatropine, scopolamine, and atropine—bolster the blood aqueous barrier, produce extended paralysis of the ciliary muscle, and inhibit the formation of posterior synechiae. Occasionally, cycloplegic drugs may be used to enhance visual function by maintaining pupillary dilation in patients with posterior subcapsular cataracts who either decline surgical extraction or have a medical contraindication to surgery.

Adverse ocular reactions include blurred vision (especially at near), hypersensitivity or toxic reactions, prolonged pupillary dilation, photophobia, and risk of elevated intraocular pressure, particularly in patients with narrow angles. Significant adverse systemic reactions include dryness of mouth, increased thirst, drowsiness, and visual hallucinations.

CLINICAL PEARL
Pupillary mydriasis may cause decreased contrast sensitivity, reduced depth of focus or field, increased chromatic and spherical aberrations, blurred vision, and increased brightness or photophobia.

Corticosteroids

Topical steroids suppress the ocular inflammatory response regardless of the underlying etiology, whether it be chemical, immunological, infectious, or traumatic. These agents are typically prescribed to treat ocular inflammatory reactions including ocular allergy, episcleritis/scleritis, uveitis, and traumatic iritis. Steroids reduce pain, redness, local heat, and swelling by reducing capillary permeability, cellular infiltration, volume of chemical mediators, mast cell degranulation, macrophage migration, and fibroblast activity. Corticosteroids also inhibit the pathways for the synthesis of prostaglandins and leukotrienes.

Steroid agents have many potentially significant adverse effects. The ocular effects include delayed corneal wound healing, elevated intraocular pressure or glaucoma, posterior subcapsular cataracts, and secondary infections. The risk for elevated intraocular pressure is frequently related to how well a particular steroid drug penetrates the cornea into the anterior chamber. Although posterior subcapsular cataracts are typically seen with systemic corticosteroid therapy, there is risk for their formation in cases of prolonged topical drug usage.

CLINICAL PEARL
All patients using topical steroids need to be closely monitored for the development of elevated intraocular pressure, cataracts, or other complications which could have a detrimental effect upon ocular health or efficient visual performance.

TABLE 5-1

Ocular Components Potentially Affected by Glaucoma Agents Which May Influence Functional Vision

Drug category	Ocular surface affected	Pupil size changed	Accomodation affected	Visual field affected	Perceived brightness	Depth of field or focus
Beta-blockers	Yes	No	No	No	No	No
Sympathomimetics	Yes	Yes	No	No	No	No
Miotics	+/−	Yes	Yes	Yes	Yes	Yes
Carbonic anhydrase Inhibitors	No	No	No	No	No	No

Glaucoma Agents

Medical management of glaucoma involves lowering the intraocular pressure by either decreasing the rate of aqueous production or increasing the rate of aqueous outflow through the trabecular meshwork. Lowering the intraocular pressure reduces the risk for optic nerve damage or loss of visual field with subsequent loss of vision. The pharmacologic actions of topical glaucoma medications (Table 5-1) can be classified into four categories: beta adrenergic blockers, adrenergic agonist (sympathomimetic) agents, miotic (cholinergic) agents, and carbonic anhydrase inhibitors.

Beta adrenergic blockers

These include the nonselective drugs, timolol, levobunolol, metipranolol, and carteolol and the cardiac selective drug betaxolol. These agents lower intraocular pressure by decreasing aqueous production. Beta adrenergic blockers may be used alone or in combination with other drugs.

These drugs may have several adverse ocular effects including dry eye syndrome, ocular surface abnormalities, corneal epitheliopathy, superficial punctate keratitis, decreased corneal sensitivity, hypersensitivity reactions, and blurred vision. Significant adverse systemic effects consist of respiratory failure, bradycardia, hypotension, depression, lethargy, and decreased sex drive. Although betaxolol has a lower risk for respiratory problems, caution should be exercised in patients at risk for asthma.

CLINICAL PEARL

Many patients using beta adrenergic blockers have significant corneal epitheliopathy which frequently results in decreased contrast sensitivity, hazy vision, and photophobia.

> ### CLINICAL PEARL
> *Subtle clinical depression following administration of topical beta adrenergic blocking agents is often overlooked by many clinicians. This may affect the patient's interest in a visual rehabilitation program or possibly complicate previously diagnosed depression related to the psychological trauma associated with loss of vision.*

Adrenergic agonist (sympathomimetic) agents

These agents include dipivefrin, epinephrine, and apraclonidine. These drugs lower intraocular pressure by decreasing aqueous production and, in the case of dipivefrin and epinephrine, possibly also by increasing aqueous outflow. They may be used alone or in combination with other medications.

Adverse ocular effects include burning or stinging upon instillation, foreign body sensation, lacrimation, hypersensitivity or toxic reactions, and mydriasis. Adverse systemic reactions for dipivefrin and epinephrine include hypertension, cardiac arrhythmias, and tachycardia. Apraclonidine may cause dry mouth or nose, cardiac arrhythmias, and depression.

> ### CLINICAL PEARL
> *When patients use a sympathomimetic drug alone or in combination with a beta adrenergic blocker they may have transient or fluctuating small changes in pupil size over several hours with subsequent blurred vision complaints while performing tasks with their optical devices.*

Miotic (cholinergic) agents

These agents can be divided into two classes: direct acting and indirect acting. Direct acting miotics are parasympathomimetic agents which produce constriction of the iris sphincter and cause the longitudinal muscle of the ciliary body to have increased tension on the scleral spur. This leads to increased aqueous outflow due to an opening of the trabecular meshwork channels. The direct acting miotics consist of pilocarpine and carbachol. Pilocarpine is the most frequently prescribed agent of all the miotics for the treatment of glaucoma.

Indirect acting miotics are cholinesterase inhibitors which potentiate the action of endogenous acetylcholine through inactivation of the enzyme acetylcholinesterase. These drugs have a longer duration of action than the direct acting miotics and may be further categorized as reversible or irreversible. The irreversible agents have the longest duration of action. Physostigmine (reversible) and echothiophate iodide (irreversible) are the most commonly utilized cholinesterase inhibitor drugs. Miotic agents may be used alone or in combination with other glaucoma drugs, particularly the beta adrenergic blockers.

These agents have several adverse ocular effects including miosis, accommodative spasm, blurred vision, brow ache, iatrogenic myopia, conjunctival congestion, stinging or burning upon instillation, and poor dark adaptation. Retinal detachment is a risk for patients with preexisting retinal breaks or degenerations. The consistency and severity of the adverse effects vary with the particular drug. Systemic adverse effects are rare.

CLINICAL PEARL

Pupillary miosis may cause variable contrast sensitivity, increased depth of focus and field, improved vision if no media opacities are present, reduced vision with media opacities on the visual axis, less chromatic or spherical aberrations, and decreased brightness.

CLINICAL PEARL

Patients using miotics should have their pupils dilated at least every year to attain partial rejuvenation of iris sphincter muscle tone and to ensure future ability to dilate the pupil for stereo optic nerve assessments, retinal examinations, and visual field analysis.

Carbonic Anhydrase Inhibitor

The carbonic anhydrase inhibitor dorzolamide reduces intraocular pressure by inhibiting the production of the aqueous by inhibiting the enzyme carbonic anhydrase with subsequent slowing of the formation of bicarbonate ions within the ciliary processes. It can be used alone or in combination with a beta adrenergic blocker.

Adverse ocular reactions include transient burning or stinging upon instillation. Although the risk for an additive effect on the known adverse systemic reactions of oral carbonic anhydrase inhibitors exists, there appears to be no other significant systemic complications.[1]

CLINICAL PEARL

Topical dorzolamide may prove to be a very efficacious drug for lowering intraocular pressure without the adverse effects of systemic carbonic anhydrase inhibitors or the adverse ocular effects of other glaucoma agents on functional visual performance.

Hypertonic/Hyperosmotic Agents

Hypertonic or hyperosmotic agents potentiate the removal of corneal edema by making the tear film hyperosmotic relative to the cornea. Sodium chloride and glucose solutions can be used to reduce chronic corneal edema found in bullous keratopathy or Fuchs' endothelial dystrophy. Glycerin is primarily used to clear corneal edema to facilitate a diagnostic gonioscopic or ophthalmoscopic examination. Sodium chloride ointments and solutions are also useful for removing corneal microcysts associated with epithelial basement membrane dystrophy or recurrent corneal erosion.

Adverse ocular effects include burning or stinging upon instillation and corneal epitheliopathy.

CLINICAL PEARL

Sodium chloride ointment usage at bedtime often eliminates the need for daily administration of solutions. This may result in better contrast sensitivity and visual acuity for patients with microcystic edema.

Systemic Medications

Antihistamine Agents

Oral antihistamines are frequently prescribed as adjunct therapy for the relief of ocular allergy signs and symptoms, especially when significant edema of the eyelids is present. Antihistamines are used to treat allergic rhinitis, sinusitis, dermatitis, urticaria and angioedema. They also are used for relief of symptoms associated with the common cold. Antihistamines competitively antagonize or block the action of histamine at the H_1-receptor sites.[2]

Adverse ocular reactions include those that are typically attributed to anticholinergic activity, such as reduced lacrimation, dry eye syndrome, pupillary mydriasis, and blurred vision. Depending on the particular drug, the most frequently encountered adverse systemic effects are transient drowsiness and sedation (Table 5-2).

TABLE 5-2

Effects of Commonly Used Oral Antihistamines Potentially Affecting Functional Vision

Drug	Anticholinergic activity	Sedative effects
Astemizole	+/–	ns[*]
Chlorpheniramine	++	+
Clemastine	+++	++
Diphenhydramine	+++	+++
Loratadine	+/–	ns
Terfenadine	+/–	ns

[*] ns—usually not significant
Modified from *Drug facts and comparisons*, St Louis, 1995, Facts and Comparisons, 1043.

CLINICAL PEARL

Small transient changes in pupil size and decreased lacrimation affecting tear film quality or wetting of the cornea can cause vague visual complaints of hazy vision which may reduce optimal functional vision with an optical device.

Antidepressant Agents

The antidepressants comprise a group of drugs that are commonly prescribed to treat clinical depression, anxiety, and sleep disturbances. Many patients who have suffered permanent loss of vision due to disease or trauma manifest signs of clinical depression and may be prescribed antidepressant agents. These drugs improve the regulation of neurotransmission in the brain by decreasing the sensitivity of the presynaptic receptor sites and increasing the sensitivity of the postsynaptic, alpha adrenergic and serotonin, receptor sites. This correction enhances the patient's recovery from the depression inducing episode.[3]

Adverse ocular reactions include those that are typically attributed to anticholinergic activity, such as dry eye syndrome, pupillary mydriasis, diplopia, and blurred vision. Occasionally, there may be a reduction in accommodation. Depending on the particular drug, the most frequently encountered adverse systemic effects are sedation and orthostatic hypotension (Table 5-3).

CLINICAL PEARL

Patients using oral medications with anticholinergic adverse effects may require therapy for dry eye or related ocular surface disease to maintain optimal functional vision with optical devices.

TABLE 5-3
Effects of Oral Antidepressants Potentially Affecting Functional Vision

Drug	Anticholinergic activity	Sedation activity
Tricyclics		
Amitriptyline	++++	++++
Clomipramine	+++	+++
Doxepin	++	+++
Imipramine	++	++
Trimipramine	++	+++
Amoxapine	+++	++
Desipramine	+	+
Nortriptyline	++	++
Protriptyline	+++	+
Phenethylamine		
Venlafaxine	−	−
Tetracyclic		
Maprotiline	++	++
Triazolopyridine		
Trazodone	+	++
Aminoketone		
Bupropion	++	++
Serotonin Reuptake Inhibitors		
Fluoxetine	+/−	+/−
Paroxetine	−	+/−
Sertraline	−	+/−

Modified from *Drug facts and comparisons,* St Louis, 1995, Facts and Comparisons, 1385.

Carbonic Anhydrase Inhibitors

The carbonic anhydrase inhibitors are nonbacteriostatic sulfonamide drugs that reduce intraocular pressure by suppressing the production of aqueous by inhibiting the enzyme carbonic anhydrase with subsequent slowing of the formation of bicarbonate ions within the ciliary processes. These agents are typically used in combination with topical glaucoma agents in cases where adequate intraocular pressure reduction could not be achieved by topical therapy alone.

Although there are no remarkable ocular adverse effects, the systemic effects are significant. Paraesthesia in the extremities, tinnitus, gastrointestinal disturbances, malaise, drowsiness, fatigue, metabolic acidosis, and electrolyte imbalances are common. Erythema multiforme, Stevens-Johnson syndrome, and hypersensitivity reactions have also been noted.[4] Treatment with oral carbonic anhydrase inhibitors is frequently discontinued due to the high incidence of these adverse effects.

CLINICAL PEARL

Patients taking oral carbonic anhydrase inhibitors may not perform as well during visual rehabilitation tasks because of chronic fatigue and general malaise symptoms.

Vitamins/Minerals

Many vitamin and mineral supplements containing vitamins A, C, and E, as well as the mineral elements selenium and zinc have been promoted for the prevention or treatment of degenerative eye diseases in recent years. Although there is strong evidence that increased dietary intake of antioxidants may lower the risk for age related macular degeneration or slow the progression of retinitis pigmentosa, the effectiveness of vitamin or mineral therapy remains controversial.

Nutritional factors may have a role in the prevention of age related macular degeneration. The National Health and Nutrition Examination Survey[5] found that patients who consume lower amounts of fruits and vegetables rich in vitamin A have a significantly higher risk for both exudative and nonexudative age related macular degeneration. The Eye Disease Case Control Study[6] confirmed this finding and also demonstrated that patients with higher plasma levels of carotenoid had a markedly reduced risk for exudative age related macular degeneration. Higher plasma levels of vitamins C and E were associated with reduced risk but the findings were statistically insignificant. The study also found that an antioxidant index, composed of plasma levels of carotenoid, vitamin C, vitamin E, and selenium, was associated with lower risk at higher values of the index. Despite this evidence, there are no conclusive data indicating that increased intake of these compounds will improve functional vision in patients who currently have age related macular degeneration. One study[7] did demonstrate that patients with age related macular degeneration retained better visual acuity with zinc supplements over a two year span than those who did not receive the supplements. However, this information has also been contradicted by data from the Eye Disease Case Control Study.[8]

A randomized trial of vitamin A and E supplements for retinitis pigmentosa found that patients taking 15,000 IU/d of vitamin A had a slower decline of retinal function as measured by the electroretinogram than patients not taking the supplement.[9] Similar trends were noted on the reduction of visual field. However, 400 IU/d of vitamin E may have an adverse effect.

Since high plasma levels of various vitamins and minerals may be toxic for some patients, the results from the ongoing National Eye Institute Age-Related Eye Disease clinical trials are still needed to adequately assess the benefits and risks of these therapies. Gastrointestinal distress including abdominal pain, nausea, and vomiting may occur with high doses of some compounds. Excessive vitamin A can be toxic to the liver and beta-carotene supplements may cause a higher mortality rate among male smokers.[10] Vitamin C is contraindicated in patients with kidney stones or hemochromatosis.[11] Vitamin E has been associated with fatigue, muscle weakness related to decreased thyroid activity, and slow blood clotting time in patients with vitamin K deficiency.[12,13] Zinc has been linked to sideroblastic anemia associated with copper deficiency, bone marrow depression, and reduced levels of high density lipoprotein cholesterol.[14,15]

CLINICAL PEARL

Vitamin and mineral supplements may be beneficial in the prevention of age related eye diseases.

CLINICAL PEARL

The patient's general medical status should be carefully evaluated before beginning any therapy with higher doses of vitamin or mineral supplements.

References

1. Package insert, Merck & Co, Inc, West Point, Pa.
2. *Drug facts and comparisons*, St Louis, 1995, Facts and Comparisons, 1043-1049.
3. *Drug facts and comparisons*, St Louis, 1995, Facts and Comparisons, 1384-1385.
4. *Drug facts and comparisons*, St Louis, 1995, Facts and Comparisons, 626-628.
5. Goldberg J, Flowerdew G, Smith E, et al: Factors associated with age-related macular degeneration: an analysis of data from the first National Health and Nutrition Examination Survey, *Am J Epidemiol* 128:700-710, 1988.
6. Antioxidant status and neovascular age-related macular degeneration, the eye disease case-control study group, *Arch Ophthalmol* 111:104-109, 1993.
7. Newsome DA, Swartz M, Leone NC, et al: Oral zinc in macular degeneration, *Arch Ophthalmol* 106:192-198, 1988.
8. A case-control study of risk factors for neovascular age-related macular degeneration, the eye disease case-control study group, *Arch Ophthalmol* 110:1701-1708, 1992.
9. Berson EL, Rosner B, Sandberg MA, et al: A randomized trial of vitamin A and vitamin E supplementation for retinitis pigmentosa, *Arch Ophthalmol* 111:761-772, 1993.
10. The effect of vitamin E and beta carotene on the incidence of lung cancer and other cancers in male smokers, the alpha-tocopherol, beta carotene cancer prevention study group, *N Engl J Med* 330:1029-1035, 1994.
11. Herbert V: Risk of oxalate stones from large doses of vitamin C, *N Engl J Med* 198:856, 1978.
12. Seddon JM, Ajani UA, Sperduto RD, et al: Dietary carotenoids, vitamins A, C, and E, and advanced age-related macular degeneration, *JAMA* 272:1413-1420, 1994.

13. Roberts HJ: Perspective on vitamin E as therapy, *JAMA* 246:129-131, 1981.

14. Broun ER, Greist A, Tricot G, Hoffman R: Excessive zinc ingestion: a reversible cause of sideroblastic anemia and bone marrow depression, *JAMA* 264:1141-1143, 1990.

15. Hooper PL, Visconti L, Garry PJ, Johnson GE: Zinc lowers high-density lipoprotein-cholesterol levels, *JAMA* 244:1960-1961, 1980.

General references

Bartlett JD, Ghormley NR, Jaanus SD, Rowsey JJ, Zimmerman TJ: *Ophthalmic drug facts,* St Louis, 1995, Facts and Comparisons.

Physicians desk reference for ophthalmology, ed 23, Montvale, NJ, 1995, Medical Economics Co.

6

A Functional Approach to the Optics of Low Vision Devices

Roy G. Cole

Key Terms

equivalent power	microscopes	reading cap
low vision aids	magnifiers	magnification
spectacles	telescopes	

Many practitioners who provide low vision care do not have a good understanding of the optical principles that apply to the low vision aids (LVAs) they and their patients are using. As a result, mistakes can be made during the examination, or during patient training with the LVA itself. The purpose of this chapter is to help the low vision practitioner develop a working knowledge of the optical principles that underlie low vision aids.

First, the concept of equivalent power will be defined and explained, and this concept will then be applied to all low vision aids used for near point tasks. The application of equivalent power to near low vision aids will help to alleviate much confusion, and it will be a unifying concept around which all near low vision aids can be categorized.

We will also look at telescopes, both distance and near, and closed-circuit televisions. A discussion of magnification will show you the problems associated with this term, and will hopefully also clear up many misconceptions about this topic. The chapter will also include practice problem sets to enable you to review and practice applying the concepts that have been discussed, and a listing of references for further elaboration of the concepts presented.

Equivalent Power

In working with the low vision patient, after the subjective testing (testing the patient's prescription) is completed, an add is predicted. What you have is now a starting point. The predicted add, with the patient's distance prescription, is placed in a trial frame and modified until the patient is reading the desired print size. The final lens is the total dioptric power of the distance prescription and the add power needed by the patient. (Note that we are assuming no accommodation by the patient at this point.) Any other aid or combination of lenses used (with or without accommodation or a spectacle add) should have a total dioptric power equivalent to this add power. Thus our approach to near low vision aids (NLVAs) is to select aids that have the same *equivalent power* (in diopters) as the add needed by the patient.

In analyzing the equivalent power of NLVAs, we know that the NLVA itself has a dioptric power (F_1), and that it can be used with or without accommodation or a reading add (both represented by a lens, F_2, located in the spectacle plane). This approach takes into account spectacle-mounted microscopes (high plus lenses), hand held magnifiers, and stand magnifiers. Near telescopes can also be specified in equivalent power, but the approach is slightly different and will be discussed separately. (Note: We consider a loupe to be a plus lens held away from the spectacle plane.)

We will be using the general relationship for equivalent power:

$$F_e = F_1 + F_2 - zF_1F_2 \qquad (1)$$

where

F_e = equivalent power (total D needed by patient)
$\quad$ (f_e = focal length of the "equivalent lens")

F_1 = power (equivalent) of the NLVA (D)
$\quad$ (f_1 = primary focal length of the NLVA)

F_2 = accommodation or add used by patient (D), represented by a plus lens positioned at the spectacle plane
$\quad$ (f_2 = primary focal length of the add, or accommodation, being used)

z = separation between the low vision aid (F_1) and the spectacle plane (location of F_2) in meters.

The clinical interpretation of equivalent power is that the whole optical system (F_1 and F_2) can be replaced by a *single lens* (F_e) positioned such that the object is located at its primary focal point. The result is parallel light leaving this lens and entering the patient's eye, a condition necessitated by the requirement of no accommodation by the patient, as discussed previously. We are assuming that the patient is emmetropic, or fully corrected. F_2 does *not* include a correction for refractive error. If it did, the refractive error would have to be added to F_2, but not considered in these calculations.

CLINICAL PEARL

The clinical interpretation of equivalent power is that the whole optical system can be replaced by a single lens positioned such that the object is located at its primary focal point.

A diagrammatic representation of Equation 1 follows (Figure 6-1). This not only shows the NLVA itself (F_1) and the spectacle add or accommodation (F_2), but also the equivalent lens (F_e) and its focal length (f_e). Note also that the image of the object created by F_1 falls at the primary focal point (f_2) of F_2 (Figure 6-2).
In addition, we can also define (see Figure 6-3)

u = object distance from F_1 *(m)*

h = eye-lens distance (vertex distance) *(m)*

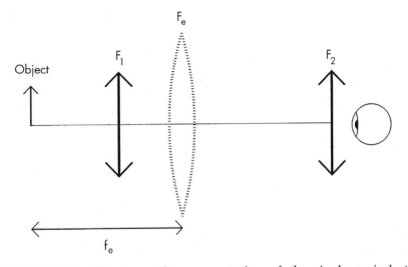

FIGURE 6-1 Diagrammatic representation of the single *equivalent* lens of a multi-lens system.

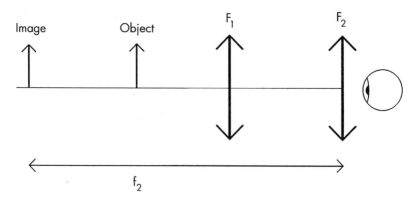

FIGURE 6-2 Image created by F_1 (of object) falls at focal point of F_2.

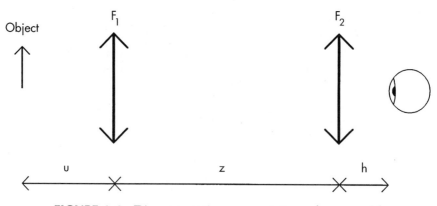

FIGURE 6-3 Diagrammatic representation of u, z, and h.

Spectacles, Hand Held Magnifiers and Stand Magnifiers

The optics of all NLVAs (telescopes will be discussed separately) can be explained by Equation 1. There are four situations that encompass their use, and we will now look at each in turn.

I.A. F_1 at Spectacle Plane, Object at f_1

In this case, since the object is at f_1, parallel light leaves F_1, and $F_2 = 0$. Thus

$$F_e = F_1 \tag{2}$$

A diagrammatic representation is given in Figure 6-4.

This case takes into account both high plus spectacles and hand held magnifiers held at the spectacle plane. The object is at the focal

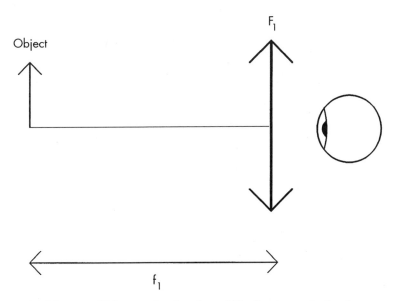

FIGURE 6-4 Object at focal point of F_1. F_1 at spectacle plane.

point of F_1, and no accommodation or add is needed. There is one other situation that can be explained here: the use of accommodation alone by, for example, a child who holds a book very close to read. In this case, $F_1 = 0$, and $F_e = F_2$.

I.B. F_1 outside Spectacle Plane, Object at f_1

In this case, since the object is at f_1, parallel light leaves F_1, and $F_2 = 0$. Thus

$$F_e = F_1 \tag{3}$$

A diagrammatic representation of this is given in Figure 6-5. Note that z is NOT = 0, but $F_2 = 0$.

  This case takes into account a hand held magnifier used away from the eye (spectacle plane) without an add or accommodation being needed. The equivalent power of this system is independent of the eye-lens distance (h), and is constant. This can be explained diagrammatically in Figure 6-6. Note that the angular subtense (θ) of the light entering the eye is the same for any value of h (h_1, h_2, or h_3), where h_1 represents situation I.A., and h_2 and h_3 represent situation I.B. Note also that Equations 2 and 3 are the same.

  One question that often arises here is "If the power (and thus the magnification) is constant irrespective of h, why does a hand held magnifier seem to magnify more at a greater distance than at a closer distance?" The answer is that the angular size of the image viewed

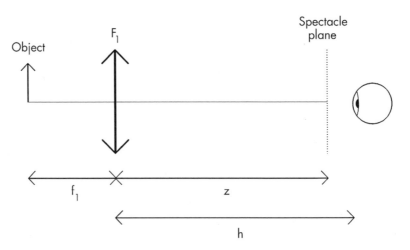

FIGURE 6-5 Object at focal point F_1. F_1 away from spectacle plane.

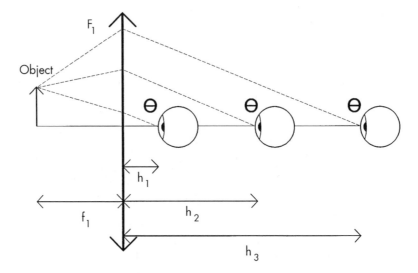

FIGURE 6-6 Angular subtense of image is same irrespective of distance between magnifier and eye.

through the lens is constant on the retina, but the angular size of the object viewed outside the magnifier (and the angular size of the magnifier itself) decreases with increased viewing distance. Thus what one perceives as additional magnification through the lens as it is moved away is actually a minification of the object viewed outside the lens. Bailey refers to this as "apparent magnification." A diagrammatic representation of this is given in Figure 6-7.

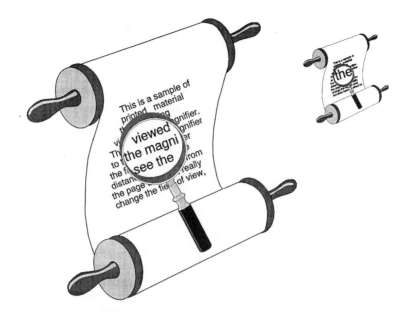

FIGURE 6-7 For a lens-page distance equal to the focal length of the magnifier, image size is constant (although it does not appear to be so), but field-of-view decreases as eye-lens distance increases.

We will examine the formulas for magnification relating to this case later. It should also be noted that the field of view through F_1 decreases with the increased distance of F_1 from the eye (h), as can also be seen in Figure 6-7.

II.A. F_1 at Spectacle Plane, Object inside f_1

In this case, since the object is inside f_1, divergent light leaves F_1 and either acommodation or an add (F_2) is required to place a clear image on the patient's retina. Thus

$$F_e = F_1 + F_2 \qquad (4)$$

A diagrammatic representation is given in Figure 6-8. Note that z = 0 in this case.

This case takes into account high plus lenses, hand held magnifiers, and stand magnifiers that are held at the eye (spectacle plane) and used in conjunction with an add or accommodation. (See II.B. for a further discussion of stand magnifiers.)

An example of this case is a patient holding a hand held magnifier against a pair of reading glasses. Another example would be a child reading at a distance closer to the eye than that predicted by the focal length of the reading lens.

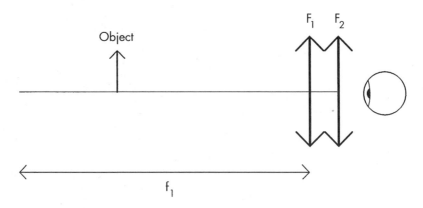

FIGURE 6-8 Object inside focal point of F_1. F_1 at spectacle plane.

II.B. F_1 outside Spectacle Plane, Object inside f_1

In this case, since the object is inside f_1, divergent light leaves F_1 and either accommodation or an add (F_2) is required to place a clear image on the patient's retina.Thus

$$F_e = F_1 + F_2 - zF_1 F_2 \tag{5}$$

A diagrammatic representation is given in Figure 6-9.

This case takes into account both hand held magnifiers and stand magnifiers held away from the eye. We will now look at each one separately.

Hand held magnifiers

One question that often arises is "Should I have the patient use the magnifier with or without a spectacle add in place?" Bailey rearranges Equation 5 to enable us to answer this question. His working equation becomes

$$Fe = F_1 - F_2 \left(\frac{z}{f_1} - 1 \right) \tag{6}$$

Analysis of this equation results in the following conclusions:

when $z = 0$	$F_e = F_1 + F_2$	Use add
when $0 < z < f_1$	$F_e > F_1$	Use add
when $z = f_1$	$F_e = F_1$	Power equality distance
when $z > f_1$	$F_e < F_1$	Use distance Rx
	$(F_2 = 0 \Rightarrow F_e = F_1)$	
when $z = f_2$	$F_e = F_2$	

So, when the distance between the spectacle plane and the hand held magnifier is less than the focal length of the magnifier (f_1), use

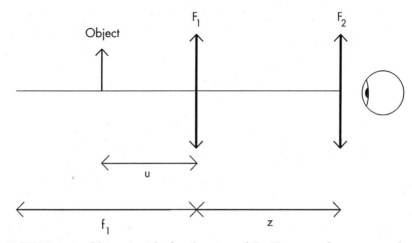

FIGURE 6-9 Object inside focal point of F_1. F_1 away from spectacle plane.

an add for maximum power. When this distance is greater than f_1, use the distance prescription alone (no add) for maximum power (same as situation I.A.). In this second case, the magnifier used with the add will actually result in less power than if the magnifier is used with no add. Note that there is an outer limit beyond which the hand magnifier *cannot* be used with the bifocal add. This outer point is the object distance being equal to the focal length of the add. At this distance, the hand magnifier must be placed *on* the object, so there is no power contribution from F_1 (also "unity magnification" results), and the total equivalent power equals the power of the add ($F_e = F_2$). This can also be seen in Equation 6 by letting $z = f_2$:

$$F_e = F_1 - F_2 \left(\frac{f_2}{f_1} - 1\right)$$

$$F_e = F_1 - \left(\frac{1}{f_2}\right)\left(\frac{f_2}{f_1}\right) + F_2$$

$$F_e = F_1 - F_1 + F_2$$

$$F_e = F_2$$

If the object is held farther than this distance, no clear erect image is possible. The only way an image could be clearly viewed would be to hold the hand magnifier in such a manner that it acts with the add as an astronomical telescope focused for near. The result would be a clear inverted image.

An example will hopefully clarify this. Consider a +20 D hand held magnifier used with +4.00 D add. Consider the following cases: (a) z = 0, (b) z = 5 cm, (c) z = 10 cm, (d) z = 25 cm, (e) z = 30 cm, and (f) z = 35 cm.

(a) $F_e = F_1 + F_2 - zF_1 F_2 = (+20) + (+4) - (0) = +24$ D
So use an add for maximum power. With F_1 used alone, $F_e = +20$ D.

(b) $F_e = (+20) + (+4) - (.05)(+20)(+4) = +20$D.
This is the same as F_1 used without an add ($F_2 = 0$), so the magnifier can be used with or without the add in this case.

(c) $F_e = (+20) + (+4) - (.1)(+20)(+4) = (+24) - (+6) = +18$D.
This is less than F_1 used alone, so you should not have the patient use an add in this case.

(d) $F_e = (+20) + (+4) - (.25)(+20)(+4) = +4$ D.
This is the same as F_2 (the add) used without a magnifier ($F_1 = 0$), so the magnifier is not helping at all.

(e) $F_e = (+20) + (+4) - (.30)(+20)(+4) = +0$ D.
The magnifier and add are acting like an afocal telescope.

(f) $F_e = (+20) + (+4) - (.35)(+20)(+4) = -4$ D.
The magnifier is actually detracting from the add power. The patient sees a smaller and inverted image.

Again, it should be noted that the farther away the magnifier is from the eye, the smaller will be the field of view through it as perceived by the patient.

Stand magnifiers—fixed focus

Although the lens-to-page distance can be varied with hand held magnifiers, this is not the case with fixed-focus stand magnifiers (variable-focus stand magnifiers, e.g., Sloane magnifiers, 15X and 20X COIL stand magnifiers, will be discussed next). Thus a slightly different approach to their analysis is required.

A fixed-focus stand magnifer (FFSM) creates a virtual image of the object, as seen in Figure 6-10. Since the object is inside f_1, divergent light leaves F_1 , and either an add or accommodation (F_2) is required to allow parallel light to enter the eye (Figure 6-11). Note: u = object distance from F_1 and u′ = image distance from F_1

The amount of accommodation or add required will depend on the position of the virtual image or, conversely, the positioning of the FFSM (and its virtual image) will depend on the add or accommodation used. Note that the image created by the stand magnifier is positioned at the focal point of the add being used. The distance of the virtual image behind the lens will also determine the maximum add that can be used.

Let us now look further at how a FFSM works. The virtual image is larger than the object in proportion to the image and object distances, i.e.,

$$MT = \text{transverse magnification}$$

$$MT = \frac{\text{image height}}{\text{object height}} = \frac{u'}{u} = \frac{U}{U'} \tag{7}$$

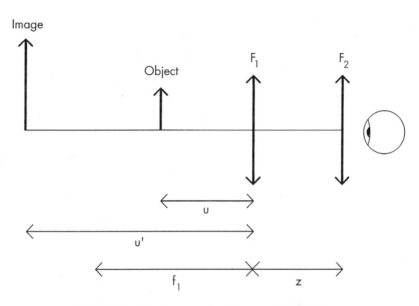

FIGURE 6-10 Image of object created by F_1.

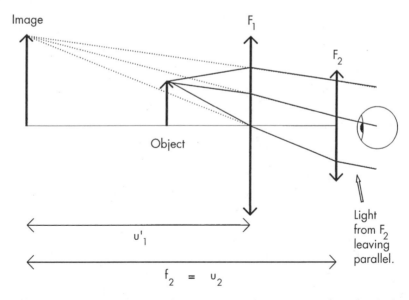

FIGURE 6-11 Image created by F_1 is at focal point of F_2 for light entering eye to have zero vergence.

Using vergence analysis:

$$U + F_1 = U'$$

$$U = U' - F_1$$

where

U = object vergence into F_1

U' = image vergence out of F_1

so

$$MT = \frac{U' - F_1}{U'} \tag{8}$$

U' can be measured by placing plus lenses over the stand magnifier until the image seen starts to blur. The last lens allowing a clear image gives us U'. F_1 can be determined with any appropriate method (see Bailey's articles in *Optometric Monthly*). Note that F_1 is an equivalent power of a thick lens, not a back vertex power, so a lensometer reading will not give a correct value. Note also that U' gives us the image location u'. Knowing the image location allows us to determine the correct position of the FFSM in front of the add (i.e., the correct z), or the amount of accommodation needed to view the image. It also allows us to calculate F_e.

We are viewing an enlarged image at some viewing distance— generally some near viewing distance requiring either an add or accommodation. The enlarged image of the object is created by the lens of the stand magnifier (Figure 6-12). The amount of enlargement (MT) times the power of the add gives us F_e. Another way to look at this is that the object would have to be moved closer to the eye by a factor of 1/MT to give us the same enlargement. The dioptric equivalent of this would be (MT)(add). Thus

$$F_e = (MT) (F_2) \tag{9}$$

Note that F_2 can be rewritten as

$$F_2 = \frac{1}{z - u'}$$

This gives us the dioptric demand if the object were placed at the image location but without the magnifier in place. So, still another way to look at MT is as the ratio of the power (F_e) used to view the image with the lens of the FFSM in place, to the power (F_2) used to view the object (placed at the location of the image) but without the lens of the FFSM in place, i.e.,

$$MT = \frac{F_e}{F_2} \tag{9a}$$

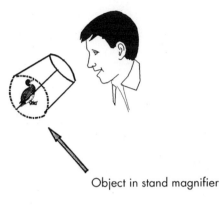

Object in stand magnifier

Image being viewed

FIGURE 6-12 Patient looking into stand magnifier is viewing enlarged image positioned away from the object.

Let's look at an example (Figure 6-13):

Let: $F_1 = +15\ D$; $F_2 = +3\ D$; and $u = -5$ cm

Since: $u = -5$ cm, $U = -20\ D$; $U' = U + F_1 = (-20) + (+15) = -5\ D$

Thus: $u' = -20$ cm

and $MT = U/U' = (-20)/(-5) = 4X$ (This is the transverse magnification of the stand magnifier.)

If a $+3\ D$ add is used (F_2), $z = 13.3$ cm = the separation between the stand magnifier's lens and the add

(since $f_2 = 33.3$ cm, and $u' = -20$ cm, then $z = f_2 + u'$)

Using Equation 9:

$$F_e = (MT)(F_2) = (4)(3) = +12\ D$$

This can also be calculated from Equation 5:

$$F_e = F_1 + F_2 - zF_1F_2$$
$$= (15) + (3) - (0.133)(15)(3)$$
$$= 18 - (0.133)(45) = 18 - 6 = +12\ D$$

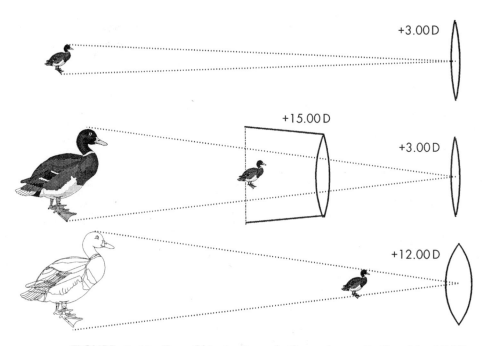

FIGURE 6-13 *Top,* Object viewed through a +3 D add. *Middle,* Enlarged image from stand magnifier positioned at the focal point of the +3 D add. *Bottom,* Object viewed through lens with same equivalent power as stand magnifier/add combination.

Note that as the add is changed, F_e changes. Once MT is known for a stand magnifier, F_e can easily be calculated for any add, as seen above. Also, in the example above, the maximum add usable is +5 D, since $u' = -20$ cm. Any add stronger than +5 D will not allow the image to be viewed clearly since the image is located outside of f_1.

Another example: A +10 D lens (F_1) is mounted 5 cm from the page (Figure 6-14, pg. 157). Wavefront analysis will show that the image is located 10 cm from the lens, i.e., 5 cm behind the page. Consider three eye-to-lens distances (z), each requiring a different add (F_2):

(a) z = 30 cm → eye-to-image = 40 cm → F_2 = +2.50 D
   $F_e = (10) + (2.50) - (.3)(10)(2.50) = +5$ D

(b) z = 15 cm → eye-to-image = 25 cm → F_2 = +4.00 D
   $F_e = (10) + (4) - (.15)(10)(4) = +8$ D

(c) z = 0 cm → eye-to-image = 10 cm → F_2 = +10.00 D
   $F_e = (10) + (10) - (0)(10)(10) = +20$ D
   Note that this is the maximum add allowable for this particular stand magnifier.

We can now see why the COIL stand magnifier labeled +28 D on the box is listed as a +17.6 D stand magnifier in the Lighthouse catalogue. The additional piece of information needed here is that the +17.6 D label is an equivalent power based on a +2.50 D add. Any other add will result in a different F_e.

Table 6-1 gives a summary of the pertinent information needed for various stand magnifiers. The following information is given in the numbered columns in this table: (1) name of magnifier; (2) manufacturer's catalogue number; (3) Lighthouse catalogue number; (4) manufacturer's labeled power; (5) "true dioptric power" (TDP) of the lens (F_1) listed in the Lighthouse catalogue; (6) power of the lens (F_1) that was measured by the author and colleagues, or previously published; (7) transverse magnification calculated from columns #6 and #9; (8) lens-to-image distance; (9) maximum add that can be used (based on emerging vergence from the lens F_1); (10) equivalent power of stand magnifier when used alone; (11) equivalent power of stand magnifier when used with a +1.00 D add; (12) equivalent power of stand magnifier when used with a +2.00 D add; (13) equivalent power of stand magnifier when used with a +2.50 D add; (14) equivalent power of stand magnifier when used with a +3.00 D add; (15) equivalent power of stand magnifier when used with a +4.00 D add; (16) equivalent power of stand magnifier when used with the maximum add listed in column #9; and (17) category based on classification used by Freed. Freed's classifications are as follows.

1. The image is at some finite distance and viewed with either an add or accommodation. The field through the magnifier is large enough that it is usually used at some distance from the eye, but also can be used at the eye (spectacle plane). In this case, the equivalent power is given by the transverse magnification (MT) times the add (or accommodation) being used [F_e = (transverse magnification) × (F_2)].

2. The image is fairly far from the magnifier, and the magnifier is designed to be used at any distance from the eye (spectacle plane) with little or no add or accommodation (i.e., with the patient's distance glasses). The equivalent power is thus approximately equal to the power of the lens itself ($F_e = F_1$).

3. The image is at some finite distance from the magnifier, and because the field is small, the magnifier should be used at the eye (spectacle plane) with the appropriate add (maximum add) in place. The equivalent power is thus the power of the stand magnifier's lens plus the power of the add ($F_e = F_1 + F_2$).

The main concept here is that the equivalent power of the stand magnifier (i.e., how it seems to the patient) depends on how it is designed to be used, and also how it is actually being used. It is this area that seems to be most confusing to students (and practitioners), and the table is designed to help understand and utilize the principles discussed in this chapter.

TABLE 6-1
Various Parameters Needed to Understand How Stand Magnifiers Are Used and Work in a Clinical Setting

(1) Name of device	(2) Manuf catalog number	(3) LH catalog number	(4) Manuf label power	(5) LH power (TDP)	(6) F_1 (D)	(7) Trans mag (X)	(8) L-1 (cm)	(9) Max add (D)	(10) No add (plo)	(11) +1.00	(12) +2.00	(13) +2.50	(14) +3.00	(15) +4.00	(16) With max add	(17) Freed cat.
									← Equivalent power of SM and add to nearest 0.25 D →							
ESCH Magnifying Rule 2D	2605	M500	1.5X	2.	30	1.3	1.	100.00	1.25	2.50	3.25	4.00	5.25	130.00	1
Selsi 6" Magnifying Rule	377	M506	3.5D	3.5	25	1.5	2.	50.00	1.50	3.00	3.75	4.50	6.00	75.00	1
B&L 6" Magna Rule	81-26-17	M504	3.5D	3.5	50	1.5	1.	100.00	1.50	3.00	3.75	4.50	6.00	75.00	1
B&L 12" Magna Rule	81-26-18	M509	3.5D	3.5	50	1.5	1.	100.00	1.50	3.00	3.75	4.50	6.00	75.00	1
Selsi Plo Cx 4.7 D	404	M515	4.7D	4.7	11	1.6	5.6	17.75	1.50	3.25	4.00	4.75	6.50	28.50	1
Selsi Plo Cx 4.7 D	403	M520	4.7D	5.	11	1.8	7.5	13.25	1.75	3.50	4.50	5.50	7.25	23.75	1
ESCH III Rect. SM 3X	1580	M546	8.0D	8.	5	1.8	15.4	6.50	1.75	3.50	4.50	5.50	7.25	11.75	1
ESCH III Rnd SM 3X	1555	M554	8.0D	8.	7	2.3	18.	5.50	2.25	4.50	5.75	7.00	9.25	12.75	1
COIL Lrg Aspheric SM 4.9D	5472	M525	8.0D	4.9	5	2.0	20.	5.00	2.00	4.00	5.00	6.00	8.00	10.00	1
COIL Bar SM 5 D	5494	M508	5.0D	8.	33	2.0	3.	33.00	2.00	4.00	5.00	6.00	8.00	66.00	1
B&L III SM 5D	81-34-80	M530	5.0D	5.	4	2.0	25.	4.00	2.00	4.00	5.00	6.00	8.00	8.00	1
COIL Hi-Power Tilt SM 3X	5213	M542	8.0D	8.	6	2.3	21.	4.75	2.25	4.50	5.75	7.00	9.25	11.00	1
COIL Small Aspheric SM	5474	M540	12.0D	8.	7	2.7	25.	4.00	2.75	5.50	6.75	8.00	10.75	10.75	1
ESCH III SM 3.4X (old 4X)	1526	M581	14.0D	13.2	12	3.2	19.	5.25	3.25	6.50	8.00	9.50	12.75	16.75	1
COIL Cat Asph SM 6X	5428	M560	20.0D	9.	16	3.3	14.8	6.75	3.25	6.50	8.25	10.00	13.50	22.25	1
ESCH III SM 4.2X (old 6X)	1525	M582	17.0D	20.	14	3.4	16.7	6.00	3.50	6.75	8.50	10.25	13.50	20.50	1
Esch SM 6X	2626	M586	20.0D	20.	15	3.5	17.	6.00	3.50	7.00	8.75	10.50	14.00	21.00	1
Selsi Jupiter SM 9 D	402	M565	9.0D	9.	12	3.9	23.5	4.25	4.00	7.75	9.75	11.75	15.50	16.50	1
COIL Rayleigh 3.9X	6259	M820	11.7D	10.8	11	4.1	29.	3.50	4.00	8.25	10.25	12.25	14.50	14.50	1
Pike III SM 5X	M5N	M590	20.0D	20.	16	6.4	33.3	3.00	6.50	12.75	16.00	19.25	-.-	19.25	1
COIL High-Power Asph SM 8X	5123	M580	28.0D	17.6	22	6.8	26.7	3.75	6.75	13.50	17.00	20.50	-.-	25.50	1
Esch SM 8X	2624	M602	28.0D	28.	21	7.1	29.	3.50	7.00	14.25	17.75	21.25	-.-	24.75	1
COIL Hi-Power Fixed SM 6X	4206	M587	20.0D	20.5	21	8.0	34.	3.00	8.00	16.00	20.00	24.00	-.-	24.00	1

TABLE 6-1 (continued)
Various Parameters Needed to Understand How Stand Magnifiers Are Used and Work in a Clinical Setting

(1)	(2)	(3)	(4)	(5)	(6)	(7)	(8)	(9)	(10)	(11)	(12)	(13)	(14)	(15)	(16)	(17)
									← Equivalent power of SM and add to nearest 0.25 D →							
Name of device	Manuf catalog number	LH catalog number	Manuf label power	LH power (TDP)	F₁ power (D)	Trans mag (X)	L-1 (cm)	Max add (D)	No add (plo)	+1.00	+2.00	+2.50	+3.00	+4.00	With max add	Freed cat.
COIL Hi-Power Tilt SM 4X	5214	M567	12.0D	11.5	12	7.9	53.	1.75	12.00	.	.	.	.	.	13.25	2
ESCH III SM 4X	1554	M570	16.0D	14.7	15	11.	67.	1.50	15.00	.	.	.	.	.	16.50	2
ESCH III SM 5X	1553	M584	20.0D	18.	19	10.5	50.	2.00	19.00	.	.	.	.	.	21.00	2
ESCH III SM 6X	1552	M585	24.0D	22.4	23	12.5	50.	2.00	23.00	.	.	.	.	.	25.00	2
ESCH III SM 7X	1551	M597	28.0D	23.4	25	13.5	50.	2.00	25.00	.	.	.	.	.	27.00	2
COIL Hi-Power SM 8X	4208	M603	28.0D	23.4	25	15.3	63.	1.75	25.00	.	.	.	.	.	26.75	2
ESCH III SM 10X	1550	M622	38.0D	40.	40	21.	50.	2.00	40.00	.	.	.	.	.	42.00	2
ESCH III SM 12.5X	1557	M608	50.0D	50.	50	23.2	44.	2.25	50.50	.	.	.	.	.	52.25	2
COIL Rayleigh 4.7X	6269	M821	14.6D	14.0	14	5.	29.	3.50		.	.	.	.	.	17.50	3
COIL Rayleigh 5.4X	6279	M822	17.7D	16.8	18	6.1	29.	3.50		.	.	.	.	.	21.50	3
COIL Rayleigh 7.1X	6289	M823	24.2D	23.1	22	6.5	25.	4.75		.	.	.	.	.	26.00	3
Pike III SM 7X	M7N	M600	28.0D	28.	26	7.9	26.7	3.75		.	.	.	.	.	29.75	3
AGFA SM 8X	AG-8	M605	33.0D	33.	28	7.6	23.5	4.25		.	.	.	.	.	32.25	3
Peak III Loupe 10X	1966	M620	40.0D	40.	29	8.7	26.7	3.75		.	.	.	.	.	32.75	3
Peak Loupe 10X	1961	M615	40.0D	40.	30	8.5	25.	4.00		.	.	.	.	.	34.00	3
COIL Hi-Power Fixed SM 10X	4210	M606	36.0D	35.	32	8.5	23.	4.25		.	.	.	.	.	36.25	3
COIL Hi-Power Fixed SM 12X	4212	M621	44.0D	44.	38	9.	21.	4.75		.	.	.	.	.	42.75	3
Peak Loupe 15X	1962	M625	60.0D	60.	46	10.7	21.	4.75		.	.	.	.	.	50.75	3
Peak III Loupe 15X	2023	M630	60.0D	45.8	46	10.2	20.	5.00		.	.	.	.	.	51.00	3
COIL Hi-Power Fixed SM 15X	4215	M626	56.0D	56.	44	4.3	14-7.5	13.25		.	.	.	.	.	57.25	3
COIL Hi-Power Fixed SM 20X	4220	M628	76.0D	65.7	55	8.8	∞-14.	7.		.	.	.	.	.	62.00	3
Peak Lupe 22X	1964	M632	22.0X	88.	67	8.8	∞	~0.		.	.	.	.	.	67.00	3

Columns 6, 7, 8, and 9 are a compilation of prior published values, actual measurements, or calculations from other variables, made by R Cole, R Rosenberg, B Freed, and K Citek.

155

> **CLINICAL PEARL**
>
> *The equivalent power of the stand magnifier (i.e., how it seems to the patient) depends on how it is designed to be used, and also how it is actually being used.*

The following are some hints on using Table 6-1.

1. If you are using a Freed Category 1 stand magnifier and know the total lens power required for the patient to read specific material, you can calculate the add required for the magnifier by dividing the total lens power by the transverse magnification (TM) of the stand. For example, a patient reads newsprint with a +15 D add, but wants to read with a 6X COIL Cataract Aspheric stand magnifier (#5428). This magnifier has a transverse magnification of 3.3. The add required would be $15/3.3 = 4.55$, so a +4.50 D add should work quite well.

2. To find the distance between the add and the stand magnifier, subtract the magnifier's lens-to-image distance from the focal length of the add being used. In the above example (in hint 1): The lens-to-add distance would be 22.2 cm (focal length of a +4.50 D add) – 14.8 cm (lens-to-image distance in the stand magnifier—column 8) = 7.4 cm, or about 7 cm. So, using the 6X stand with a +4.50 D add, and holding it about 3 inches (7+ cm) from the add should allow the patient to read the newspaper. Another example: the COIL Small Aspheric Stand magnifier (#5472) has a lens-to-image distance of 25 cm. If used with a +2.50 D add (40 cm focal length), the separation of the lens of the magnifier from the eye (add) should be $40 - 25 = 15$ cm.

3. If you know the total equivalent power of the lens required for a specific task, find that value, or one just a little less, in columns 10 - 16. For a category 1 stand magnifier, you can read the magnifier to use and the add to use. For category 2 or 3, you can read the magnifier to use, and from our previous discussions, should know how to use the magnifier in this situation.

Let's look at why labeling, or describing, stand magnifiers by only the power of the lens in the magnifier can be quite deceiving, and give results inconsistent with expected patient performance. Five stand magnifiers have been designed for this exercise (Figures 6-14, 6-15, 6-16, 6-17, and 6-18). The first three use a lens of +10.00 D, and could thus be labeled either "+10 D", "2.5X", or "3.5X"—depending on the definition of magnification chosen (see the discussion of magnification later in this chapter). The last two use a lens of +20 D, and thus could be labeled "+20 D", "5X", or "6X".

As we have seen, the magnification (TM) of the stand magnifier is a function of both the lens power and the relation of the lens to the

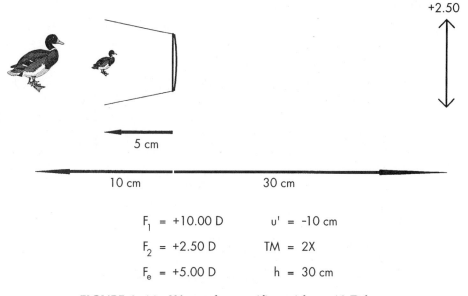

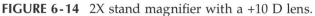

$$F_1 = +10.00 \text{ D} \qquad u' = -10 \text{ cm}$$

$$F_2 = +2.50 \text{ D} \qquad TM = 2X$$

$$F_e = +5.00 \text{ D} \qquad h = 30 \text{ cm}$$

FIGURE 6-14 2X stand magnifier with a +10 D lens.

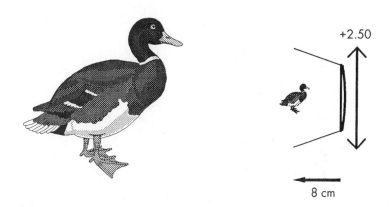

$$F_1 = +10.00 \text{ D} \qquad u' = -40 \text{ cm}$$

$$F_2 = +2.50 \text{ D} \qquad TM = 5X$$

$$F_e = +12.50 \text{ D} \qquad h = 0 \text{ cm}$$

FIGURE 6-15 5X stand magnifier with a +10 D lens.

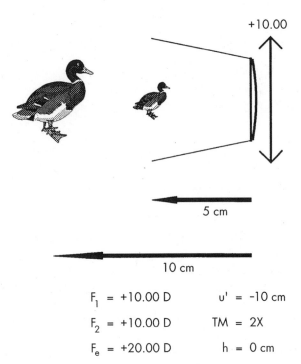

$F_1 = +10.00 \, D$ $u' = -10 \, cm$

$F_2 = +10.00 \, D$ $TM = 2X$

$F_e = +20.00 \, D$ $h = 0 \, cm$

FIGURE 6-16   2X stand magnifier with a +10 D lens.

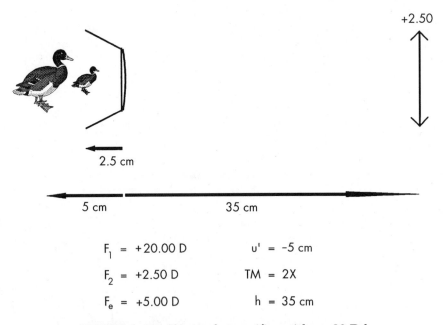

$F_1 = +20.00 \, D$ $u' = -5 \, cm$

$F_2 = +2.50 \, D$ $TM = 2X$

$F_e = +5.00 \, D$ $h = 35 \, cm$

FIGURE 6-17   2X stand magnifier with a +20 D lens.

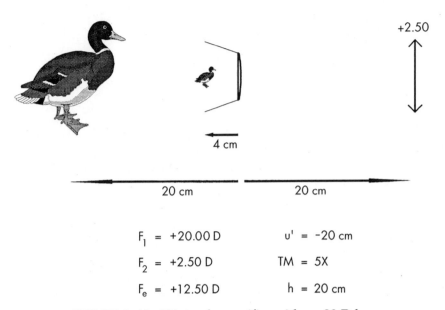

$$F_1 = +20.00 \, D \qquad u' = -20 \, cm$$

$$F_2 = +2.50 \, D \qquad TM = 5X$$

$$F_e = +12.50 \, D \qquad h = 20 \, cm$$

FIGURE 6-18 5X stand magnifier with a +20 D lens.

object (object distance/vergence vs. image distance/vergence). In the case of the stands with the +10 D lens, two magnifications have been designed: 2X (Figures 6-14 and 6-16) and 5X (Figure 6-15). The stands with the +20 D lens also have magnifications of 2X (Figure 6-17) and 5X (Figure 6-18).

As we have also seen, the equivalent powers of the stand magnifiers are a function of the magnification (TM) and the add with which the magnifier is being used. Thus depending on the add and how it is being used (distance from the stand magnifier), the three magnifiers with the +10 D lens can have equivalent powers of +5.00 D (Figure 6-14), +12.50 D (Figure 6-15), and +20.00 D (Figure 6-16). The two magnifiers with the +20 D lens can have equivalent powers of +5.00 D (Figure 6-17) and +12.50 D (Figure 6-18).

It is interesting to note that the magnifier with the weaker lens and lower magnification can have the stronger equivalent power, depending on how it is being used. Thus a magnifier with a +10 lens and 2X magnification can have a +20 D equivalent power when used with a +10.00 D add, the maximum add (Figure 6-16), while a magnifier with a +20 D lens and 5X magnification can have a +12.50 D equivalent power when used with a +2.50 D add (Figure 6-18). Also note that two magnifiers with the same magnification (TM – 5X) and the same add (+2.50) will have the same equivalent power (+12.50 D), even though the lenses have different powers (+10 D in Figure 6-15 and +20 D in Figure 6-18). Of course, the stand magnifier with the highest magnification and strongest lens, when used with the maximum add, will give the largest equivalent power. In the case of our examples, the 5X stand with the +20 D lens (Figure 6-18) when used with a +5 D add (maximum add based on -20 cm image distance) will give an equivalent power of $+25$ D. This power is also equal to the sum of the lens power in the stand magnifier and the power of the add (added together since the lenses are "touching").

Stand magnifiers—variable focus

Variable focus stand magnifiers (VFSM) are generally of higher power and designed to be used close to the eye. The lens (F_1) can be focused closer to or farther from the page so as to vary the vergence of the light leaving the lens and entering the patient's eye. VFSMs can be used with or without a spectacle add, depending on how they are focused, and situations I.B. and I.A., respectively, would apply here.

Telescopes

Before discussing near telescopes (telescopes modified for close viewing distances), a brief review of the optics of afocal telescopes is in order.

Recall the two basic types of telescopes (Figures 6-19 and 6-20).

where

f_{ep} = eyepiece focal length

f_{ob} = objective focal length

Note that the image is inverted in a Keplerian telescope, so erecting lenses or prisms are required to make it a terrestrial telescope.

Magnification for an afocal telescope is given by

$$M = -\frac{F_{ep}}{F_{ob}} = -\frac{f_{ob}}{f_{ep}} \tag{10}$$

Magnification of a focal telescope is given by

$$M = \left(\frac{1}{1 - dF_{ob}}\right)\left(\frac{1}{1 - hF_v}\right) \tag{11}$$

where

F_v = back vertex power of telescope

F_{ob} = objective lens power (F_{ep} = eyepiece power)

d = distance between objective and eyepiece = $f_{ob} + f_{ep}$

h = distance from ocular lens to eye (vertex distance)

For an afocal telescope ($F_v = 0$):

$$M = \left(\frac{1}{1 - dF_{ob}}\right) \tag{12}$$

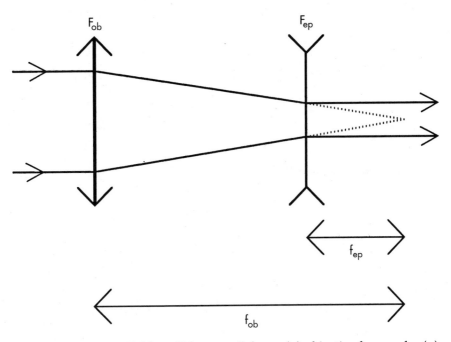

FIGURE 6-19 Galilean Telescope. It has a (+) objective lens and a (−) eyepiece.

Combining equations 10 and 12, we can see that

$$F_{ob} = \frac{M - 1}{Md} \tag{13}$$

$$F_{ep} = \frac{-F_{ob}}{1 - dF_{ob}} \tag{14}$$

Note that these formulas apply to both Keplerian and Galilean telescopes. Also note that if the patient has a refractive error, the correcting lens must be placed *behind* the telescope so as not to change focus or the power of the telescope (i.e., to leave the telescope afocal).

If the patient is ametropic and not using a spectacle correction, the telescope must be focused for the distant object. What in effect is happening is that "part" of the ocular lens is being used to compensate for the patient's ametropia, and the "balance" is now acting as the ocular of the telescope. The tube length must be adjusted to keep the telescope acting as though afocal. If the patient is a hyperope, plus (+) power is subtracted from the ocular. If the patient is a myope, minus (−) power is subtracted from the ocular. What results is that the patient is looking through a telescope that has a different magnification than the labeled value. An example should help to make this clear.

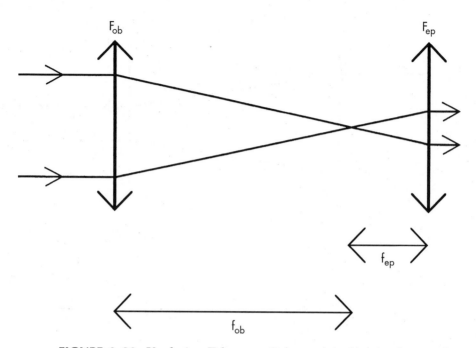

FIGURE 6-20 Keplerian Telescope. It has a (+) objective lens and a (+) eyepiece.

Example (Figure 6-21): Consider a 2X afocal Galilean telescope with a +8.00 D objective lens. From the previous discussion, we know that the ocular lens must be −16.00 D. The tube length is 6.2 cm. Let's consider what happens when an uncorrected 4.00 D hyperope uses the telescope for distance spotting. +4.00 D of the ocular must act as a correction lens, so the ocular has an effective power of −20.00 D (i.e., the −20.00 D ocular combined with the +4.00 D correction lens gives us the −16.00 D ocular the telescope actually has). To make this telescope act as though afocal, the tube length must be increased to 7.5 cm, and the telescope now has a power of 2.5X. If an uncorrected 4.00 D myope uses the telescope, −4.00 D of the ocular must act as a correction lens, so the ocular now has an effective power of −12.00 D (i.e., the −12.00 D ocular combined with the −4.00 D correction lens gives us the −16.00 D ocular the telescope actually has). To make this telescope act as though afocal, the tube length must be decreased to 4.2 cm, and the telescope now has a power of 1.5X.

When viewing a near object through an afocal telescope, the telescope acts as a vergence multiplier. The accommodation required is given by

$$A_{oc} = \frac{M^2 U}{1 - dMU} \qquad (15)$$

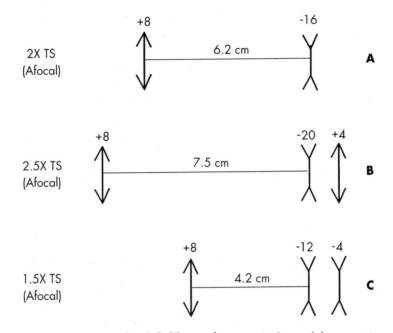

FIGURE 6-21 A 2X afocal Galilean telescope: **A,** focused for emmetrope. **B,** focused for 4 D hyperope. **C,** focused for 4 D myope.

A_{oc} can be approximated by

$$A_{oc} \approx M^2 \, U \tag{16}$$

where

A_{oc} = vergence at eyepiece = "accommodation"

U = object vergence at objective = $1/u$

Note that M is (+) for Galilean telescopes and (−) for Keplerian telescopes when used in the equations. Also, U is a negative number in these equations.

Example: A 2X Galilean telescope (+25 D objective, −50 D eyepiece) is used to view an object 40 cm from the objective lens. How much accommodation is required by the patient? There are two ways one can solve this problem:

(1) Using vergences (assuming thin lenses):
The result is that 9.1 D of accommodation is required, assuming the patient's eye is at the ocular of the telescope (Figure 6-22).

(2) Using formulas:

$$A_{oc} = \frac{M^2 \, U}{1 - dMU} = \frac{(2)^2 \, (-2.50)}{1 - (.02) \, (2) \, (-2.50)} = \frac{-10}{1.1} = -9.1 \, D$$

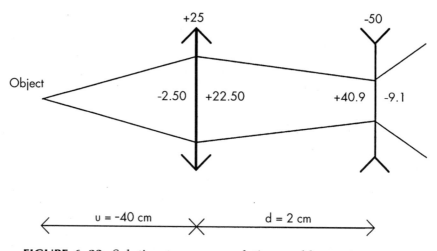

FIGURE 6-22 Solution to accommodation problem using vergence analysis.

By approximate formula:

$$A_{oc} \approx M^2\, U = -10\text{ D (i.e., 10 D of accommodation)}$$

How can we compensate for this vergence multiplication effect? There are three ways:

(1) Increase the power of the objective, or use a plus lens in front of the objective (reading cap = RC) so that the light entering the telescope will be parallel (zero vergence). In the preceding example, a +2.50 D RC is needed. The power of the reading cap is the dioptric equivalent (but opposite sign) of the object distance from F_{ob}.

(2) Decrease the ocular lens power, or use a plus lens behind the telescope. Using the same example, a +9.1 D lens applied to the back of the telescope will result in light leaving the lens with zero vergence. We could also make the ocular −40.9 D. Note that a larger amount of plus is needed behind the telescope than in front of it. It is much easier to calculate the power of a reading cap, since it is only based on the object distance from the objective lens.

(3) Increase d (separation between F_{ob} and F_{ep}). In the example, if d is increased from 2 cm to 2.44 cm, the emerging wavefront will be plano in vergence.

Equivalent Power of a Near Telescope (Using a Reading Cap Compared to Focusing)

The equivalent power of a telescope combined with a reading cap is given by

$$F_e = (F_{RC})\text{ (power of telescope)} \tag{17}$$

Example: A 3x telescope with a +4 D RC has an equivalent power of +12 D, and will enable the patient to read the same print as a +12 D add. This can also be worked in reverse. A patient needs a +12 D add to read with, but needs a 25 cm working distance. The working distance determines the reading cap power (+4 D), so +12/+4 = 3X, which is the power of the telescope needed to give a +12 D equivalent power.

Or: The patient needs +12 D to read, and already has a 3X telescope. The power of the cap needed is simply +12/3 = +4 D. Note that the working distance is increased by a factor equal to the power of the telescope when comparing a telescope/reading cap to a plus lens with the same equivalent power. It should also be noted that the depth of field is the same with the near telescope as with a spectacle lens of the same equivalent power, but the field of view is smaller.

It is important to be aware that an afocal telescope that has been focused for a close working distance does not have the same "power" (or field) as the same afocal telescope used with a reading cap that is designed for the same working distance. We have already dealt with the telescope/cap combination. Let's now look at a telescope focused for near, and see how it compares to the telescope/cap combination (Figure 6-23).

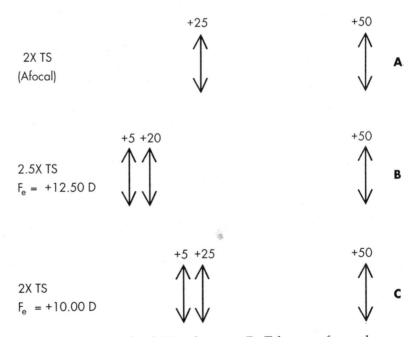

FIGURE 6-23 **A,** Afocal 2X telescope. **B,** Telescope focused on an object 20 cm away from objective. **C,** Telescope with reading cap for object 20 cm away from objective.

CLINICAL PEARL

An afocal telescope that has been focused for a close working distance does not have the same "power" (or field) as the same afocal telescope used with a reading cap that is designed for the same working distance.

The easiest way to think of this situation is to consider part of the objective lens as acting as a reading cap (Figure 6-23). The power of this "cap" is based on the distance of the object of regard. As a telescope is focused for a closer viewing distance, more and more of the objective lens is acting as the cap. This leaves a weaker objective lens for the telescope. To keep the telescope acting as though it were afocal, the tube length has to be increased. Recall that the distance between the objective lens and eyepiece on an afocal telescope equals the sum of the focal lengths of these lenses. As the objective lens becomes weaker, its focal length increases, and the separation between lenses also increases (i.e., the tube length increases). Thus the power of the telescope (M) also increases, since the power of the objective lens is less. The equivalent power of this system also increases [$F_e = (F_{cap})(M)$], and is larger than the original afocal telescope with the same cap. The field of this system is also smaller. One can now see the reason for prescribing a cap for a focusable telescope—to give the patient a larger field (albeit with less magnification) at the same working distance.

Magnification

Traditionally, magnification was taught as being one of three types: (1) relative distance magnification, which occurs when an object is brought closer to the eye, (2) relative size magnification, which occurs when the object is made larger, or (3) angular magnification, which occurs when the object is not changed in position or size, but an optical system is interposed between the object and the eye to make the object appear larger. Examples of these would be, respectively, reading glasses (the object is "enlarged" because it is brought closer to the eye with an increase in lens power), large print books, and a telescope or hand held magnifier. It is interesting to note that glasses do not magnify by themselves, but do so because the object is positioned closer to the eye.

More generally, magnification is the ratio of the angular subtense of the image viewed with the optical system to the angular subtense of the object viewed without the optical system (Figure 6-24).

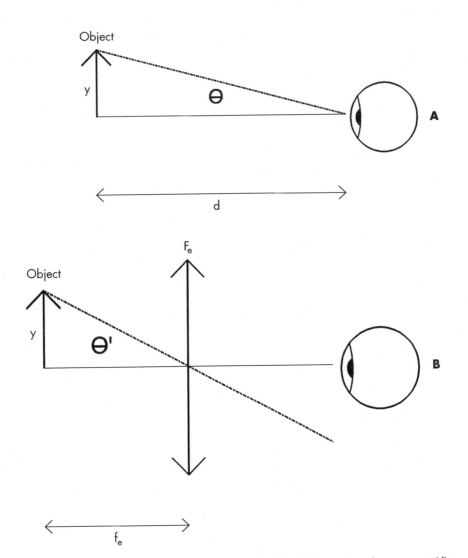

FIGURE 6-24 Angular subtense of object viewed without magnifier (**A**) and through equivalent lens of magnification system (**B**).

$$M = \frac{\theta'}{\theta} = \frac{y/f_e}{y/d} = \frac{d}{f_e} = dF_e$$

(Note: Tan $\theta \approx \theta$, where θ is in radians)
  Thus:

$$M = dF_e \qquad \text{Effective Magnification} \qquad (18)$$

where

$$d = \text{reference distance } (m)$$

Note that the object will always be at the focal point of the equivalent lens (optical system), where F_e is determined by Equation 1. The image produced by this equivalent lens (optical system) is what is viewed by the patient, and it is the angular size of this image that is compared to the angular size of the object, when the object is placed at some arbitrary distance d.

We will now look at each of the four situations discussed previously.

I.A. F_1 at Spectacle Plane, Object at f_1

$$M = dF_1 \tag{19}$$

This compares the angular size of the image formed by the lens (F_1) at infinity with the angular size of the object placed at d.

$$\text{If } d = 25 \text{ cm} \quad M = F_1/4 \tag{19a}$$

$$\text{If } d = 40 \text{ cm} \quad M = F_1/2.50 \tag{19b}$$

Note that d is a variable that can be assigned any value. Traditionally the value 25 cm was assigned to it. It was assumed that an individual could accommodate up to 4 diopters when doing close work, and so everything was based on this "least distance of distinct vision." When d = 25 cm, we have the rated magnification of F_1 :

$$M = \frac{F_1}{4} \quad \text{Rated Magnification}$$

I.B. F_1 outside Spectacle Plane, Object at f_1

The same relationships apply as in situation I.A.

$$M = dF_1$$

It should be noted that the same magnification occurs for a given reference distance irrespective of the eye-to-lens distance (h). The magnification is always based on the angular size of the object when the object is positioned at the reference distance (d).

If we want to compare the image size to the size of the object at its actual physical location, we then let d become a "variable" such that $d = f_1 + h$ (Figure 6-25).

$$M_a = dF_1 = (f_1 + h) F_1$$

and

$$M_a = 1 + hF_1 \tag{20}$$

This is referred to as angular, apparent, or perceived magnification, and gives the ratio of the image size to the object size—*at whatever distance the object is located*. Thus M_a increases with increased object distance while the effective magnification ($M = dF_e$) remains constant

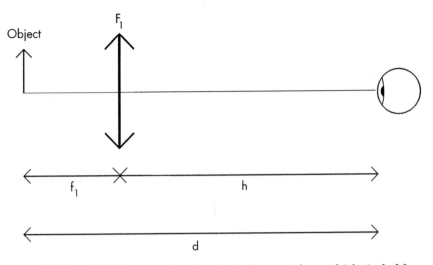

FIGURE 6-25 Object at focal point of magnifier, which is held a distance h away from the eye.

for a specific reference distance d. Refer back to the discussion of spectacles, handheld magnifiers, and stand magnifiers for further explanations and diagrams.

Note that a special case occurs when $(f_1 + h) = 25$ cm = d. We then get the rated magnification of F_1, and this is the same as $M = F_1/4$. An example will serve to demonstrate this. Consider a +20 D handheld magnifier (F_1). For an object to be 25 cm from the eye, h must be 20 cm, since $f_1 = 5$ cm (Figure 6-26).

But: $\qquad\qquad\qquad M = dF_1$ where $d = .25\ m$

Thus: $\qquad\qquad\quad M = (.25)(20) = 20/4 = 5X$

Another way to look at M_a is that it is the ratio of the total dioptric power used when viewing an object with F_1 to the power used when viewing the object without F_1 (namely, the dioptric demand of the object itself).

$$\text{Apparent Magnification} = \frac{\text{Diopters with } F_1}{\text{Diopters without } F_1} \qquad (21)$$

Consider an object at 40 cm viewed with a +10 D lens (object at the focal point of the lens):

Diopters "with" = +10   Diopters "without" = +2.50

$$M_a = \frac{+10}{+2.50} = 4X$$

The same object held at 25 cm and viewed with the same +10 D lens, would give

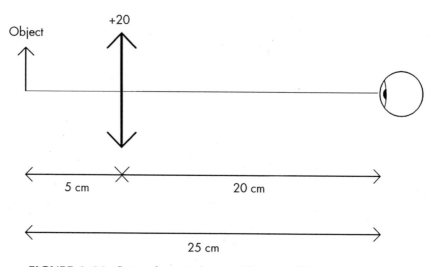

FIGURE 6-26 Setup for rated magnification. Object is positioned 25 cm in front of the eye.

$$\text{Diopters "with"} = +10 \quad \text{Diopters "without"} = +4$$

$$M_a = \frac{+10}{+4} = 2.5X$$

We can thus see that M_a increases with increased viewing distance, as was demonstrated previously.

II.A. F_1 at Spectacle Plane, Object inside f_1

$$M = d(F_1 + F_2) \tag{22}$$

In this case, the image formed by F_1 falls at some finite distance (f_2), and is "examined" by F_2.

A special case occurs when the image formed by F_1 falls at d (the reference distance). In this case, either accommodation or an add with power $F_2 = 1/d$ is required to view the image. Equation 22 then becomes

$$M_c = dF_1 + 1 \quad \text{Conventional Magnification} \tag{23}$$

and is referred to as conventional magnification. The underlying assumption here is that the patient is "supplying" one unit (1×) of magnification.

II.B. F_1 outside Spectacle Plane, Object inside f_1

Once one calculates F_e (as discussed previously), one can calculate M by

$$M = dF_e = d(F_1 + F_2 - zF_1 F_2) \tag{24}$$

In this case, the image formed by F_1 falls at some finite distance (f_2), and is "examined" by F_2. Note that the "M" value of a stand magnifier should be stated with the reference distance (or add) for which it was calculated. Unfortunately, this is usually not done.

Specifying Magnification

A question that can be posed is "How should we specify magnification in communications with other people?" The answer will vary, depending on with whom you are communicating.

If you are writing to a fellow vision care practitioner, then using the equivalent power of the system, in diopters, would be appropriate. The labeled magnification can be specified, but the dioptric equivalent should also be included. For example: "COIL 5X Hand Magnifier (+20 D)."

If you are writing to someone and want to use general terms of magnification, then it would probably be most appropriate to use angular magnification, since it represents the subjective enlargement noted by the patient better than any other definition of magnification. An example would be "6X Eschenbach hand magnifier, giving the student approximately a 4 times enlargement of his reading material," or perhaps just saying "An Eschenbach hand magnifier. . ." to avoid the confusion that might result from giving two different magnification values of the same lens. This would apply, for example, to a +20 D hand magnifier being used to look at print which is 8 inches away. The "diopters without" is +5 D, and the "diopters with" is +20 D, giving an apparent magnification of 4X (20/5). In this case, one could say that "The patient is using a handheld magnifier which gives him 4X enlargement at his customary reading distance of 8 inches."

A Final Note on Magnification

A problem can occur when using "magnification" to specify the power of a low vision device. Namely, one does not necessarily know which definition of magnification is being used. Today, some companies use F/4, some use (F/4 + 1), and one company is currently converting its labeling from (F/4 + 1) to F/4. It is important to know how the company determined the magnification listed on the box, or on the magnifier itself. Using diopters would avoid this confusion. We only have one definition for diopter. Thus we know that both hand magnifiers are the same when labeled +20 D, but one has a box labeled 5X while the other is in a box labeled 6X. It is very important to note that this whole area of magnification is defined in the ANSI-OLA Z80.9-1993 American National Standards for Ophthalmics - Low Vision Aids. It is incumbent upon all of us to know the standards, and to insist that all companies making low vision devices comply with the standards. Based on this discussion, one can now see why my talk on magnification is sometimes subtitled: "Magnification Should Be An X-Rated Subject."

> **CLINICAL PEARL**
>
> *This whole area of magnification is defined in the ANSI-OLA Z80.9-1993 American National Standards for Ophthalmics - Low Vision Aids. It is incumbent upon all of us to know the standards, and to insist that all companies making low vision devices comply with the standards.*

Equivalent Power of a CCTV

One can approximate the equivalent power of a closed-circuit television (CCTV) by considering that it uses a combination of relative size magnification (enlarging the letters) and relative distance magnification (viewing the enlarged letters at some specific distance from the screen). The relation giving the equivalent power can be written as

$$F_e = (F_2) \text{ (enlargement factor)} \tag{25}$$

where the enlargement factor is the actual physical enlargement of the object onto the video screen. For example, if a CCTV has an image on the screen 5X larger than the object, and it is viewed with a +4.00 D add, the equivalent power is $(5) \times (4) = 20$ D (i.e., the patient should theoretically be able to read the same with the +20 D add as with the CCTV at this setting).

> **CLINICAL PEARL**
>
> *One can approximate the equivalent power of a closed-circuit television (CCTV) by considering that it uses a combination of relative size magnification and relative distance magnification.*

Field of View of a Magnifier with u = f₁

One topic I would like to include is a discussion of the field of view of a magnifier with $u = f_1$:

$$W = A \left(\frac{f_1}{h} \right) \tag{26}$$

where

W = linear width of field seen through magnifier

A = linear width of the magnifying lens

f_1 = focal length of magnifying lens

h = eye-to-lens distance

Thus:

(a) If the eye is one focal length (f_1) away from the magnifier ($f_1 = h$), then the field of view is equal to the width of the lens.

(b) If the eye is only $1/2\ f_1$ from the magnifier ($f_1/h = 2$), the field of view will be equal to twice the lens diameter.

(c) If the eye is 2 f_1 from the magnifier ($f_1/h = 0.5$), the field of view would be equal to one-half the lens diameter.

References

American National Standards for Ophthalmics - Low Vision Aids, ANSI-OLA Z80.9-1993, Merrifield, Va, Optical Laboratories Association.

Bailey IL: Locating the image in stand magnifiers, *Optom Month* 72(6): 22-24, 1981.

Bailey IL: Verifying near vision magnifiers, part I, *Optom Month* 72(1): 42-43, 1981. part II, *Optom Month* 72(2): 342D37, 1981.

Bailey IL: Magnification for near vision, *Optom Month* 71:119-122, 1980.

Bailey IL: Combining accommodation with spectacle additions, *Optom Month* 71:397-399, 1980.

Bailey IL: Combining hand magnifiers with spectacle additions, *Optom Month* 71:458-461, 1980.

Bailey IL: Prescribing low vision reading aids—a new approach, *Optom Month* 72(7): 6-8, 1981.

Cole R: A unified approach to the optics of low vision aids, part I, *J Vis Rehabil* 2(1): 23-36, 1988.

Cole R: A unified approach to the optics of low vision aids, part II, *J Vis Rehabil* 2(2): 45-54, 1988.

Cole R: A unified approach to the optics of low vision aids, part III, *J Vis Rehabil* 2(4): 69-79, 1988.

Fannin T, Grosvenor T: *Clinical optics,* Boston, 1987, Butterworth.

Faye E: *Clinical low vision,* ed 2, Boston, 1984, Little, Brown & Co.

Freed B: A new method of the measurement of transverse magnification: initial results in 21 selected stand magnifiers, *J Vis Rehabil* 1(2): 47-56, 1987.

Freed B: Clinical categories of stand magnifiers, *J Vis Rehabil* 4(1): 49-52, 1990.

Mehr E, Freid A: *Low vision care,* Chicago, 1975, The Professional Press, Inc.

Newman J: *A guide to the care of low vision patients,* Missouri, 1974, American Optometric Association.

Rosenthal BP, Cole RG (eds): *Problems in optometry: a structured approach to low vision,* Philadelphia, 1991, Lippincott.

Acknowledgement

I would like to thank the following individuals: Bruce Rosenthal, who has listened to me lecture on this material many times, and who has provided good comments, encouragement, and support; Ian Bailey, who initially published and pushed many of the concepts used in this chapter; Bob Rosenberg, Alan Innes, and Ben Freed, for reading and critiquing this material, and helping me to clarify my explanations on some of the concepts discussed; and Kathy Allen-Aquilante for helping to write and check the problem sets.

Appendix: Problems

Note: Unless otherwise stated, all patients are assumed to be em-
metropes and absolute presbyopes.

Equivalent Power

1. A +10.00 D lens is used with a +5.00 D lens. What is the
   equivalent power of the system if the lens separation is (a) 20
   cm, (b) 15 cm, (c) 10 cm, (d) 0 cm?

Spectacles, Hand Magnifiers, Stand Magnifiers

2. A patient reads with a +10.00 D AOlite lens, holding the book
   10 cm from the lens. What is the equivalent power of the lens?
3. A +6.00 D spectacle lens is used by a 15-year-old emmetropic
   patient to view an object 10 cm in front of the spectacle plane.
   Assuming the object is seen clearly, what is the equivalent
   power of the eye-lens system the patient is using?
4. A young child reads a book held 5 cm from her eyes. (a) What
   is the equivalent power of her reading effort? (b) What if she
   wears a +10 D sphere and reads at 5 cm?
5. A young child has +4.00 D reading glasses, but holds the book
   at 10 cm. (a) What is the total equivalent power of his reading
   effort? (b) How much accommodation is he supplying?
6. A +8.00 D spectacle reading lens is *held* by the patient to read a
   stove setting. The lens-to-dial distance is 12.5 cm. The lens-to-
   eye distance is 37 cm. What is the equivalent power of the lens
   for this patient?
7. A patient holds his +12.00 D hand magnifier up against his
   +2.50 D add bifocal segment for reading. What is the equivalent
   power of this magnifier/bifocal system?
8. A +16 D hand held magnifier is held in front of a +2.50 D add with
   10 cm distance between the two lenses. An object held in front of
   the hand magnifier is viewed clearly through the system. What is
   the equivalent power of this magnifier/bifocal system?
9. A patient uses a +20.00 D hand magnifier with bifocals that
   have a +2.50 D add. When the hand magnifier is held 25 cm
   from the glasses, what is the equivalent power of the
   magnifier/bifocal system when the patient looks (a) above the
   bifocal segment, and (b) through the bifocal segment? (c) At
   what distance is $F_e = F_1$?
10. A patient is using a +6.00 D hand magnifier to do a number of
    tasks: (a) check stove settings at 18 inches, (b) read a computer
    screen at 16 inches, and (c) read the TV page at $4\frac{1}{2}$ inches. He has
    bifocal glasses with a +3.00 D add. How should the patient be told
    to use the hand magnifier with his glasses for the various tasks
    listed so that he benefits from the maximum power possible?

11. A patient brings in a stand magnifier that you have never seen before. You measure the equivalent power of the lens, and find it to be +10.00 D. The image formed by the stand magnifier is found to be 50 cm below the plane of the lens. (a) What is the enlargement factor for this magnifier? The patient is using the stand magnifier with glasses that have a power equivalent to a +3.50 D add. (b) What is the equivalent power of the stand magnifier with these glasses?

12. A patient can read the want ads in the local paper with a +24.00 D add. He is unhappy, however, with the close viewing distance. You prescribe a stand magnifier that enlarges everything 6X, and creates the enlarged image 20 cm behind the lens of the magnifier. What add should this patient use with the stand magnifier, and how far away should he hold the magnifier from his glasses, to get the same resolution capability that he had with the high add?

13. A patient selects a 6X COIL Cataract Aspheric Stand Magnifier (#5428). It will be used with a +3.00 D add. What distance should the stand magnifier be held from the add (spectacle plane)? What equivalent power will the patient experience when using this stand/add combination? (See Table 1 for pertinent information.)

Telescopes

14. An afocal Keplerian telescope has an objective lens that is +7.00 D and an eyepiece that is +17.50 D. What is the separation between the lenses? What is the power of the telescope?

15. A 3X afocal Galilean telescope has a separation between its lenses of 6.67 cm. What is the power of the objective and the ocular lenses?

16. A patient uses a focusable 2X Keplerian telescope that has a +8.00 D objective lens. What is the power and tube length of the afocal telescope when used by an emmetropic patient and focused for distance viewing? When used by a 4.00 D hyperope in a similar fashion? When used by a 4.00 D myope in a similar fashion? (See text for a discussion of the focusable Galilean telescope, and compare the effect on power when used by patients with various refractive errors.)

17. A patient views an object 33 cm in front of an afocal Keplerian telescope which is made up of a +20.00 D objective lens and a +40.00 D ocular lens. How much accommodation is required? (Use exact formula, not the approximate formula.)

18. A focusable Galilean telescope with a +20.00 D objective lens and a −40.00 D ocular lens is dispensed to a patient for a variety of tasks. (a) What is the magnification of this telescope at distance? (b) What tube length is required for viewing distant

objects? (c) What is the tube length required for viewing numbers that are 20 inches away in an elevator?

19. A 3X afocal Galilean telescope has a separation between the objective and ocular lenses of 2 cm. (a) What is the accommodative demand when viewing an object 25 cm away through this telescope? (b) What power reading cap would eliminate the need to accommodate for this target distance?

20. An emmetropic patient needs a 10 D add to read the text on a computer monitor, but the 10 cm working distance is too close. He wants to work at a 25 cm distance. What theoretical telescope and reading cap combination would be needed?

21. What is the equivalent lens that should be prescribed to replace a 4X telescope with a +2.50 D reading cap so the patient has the same resolution ability through the lens that he has through the telemicroscopic system?

22. If a patient is able to read enlarged sheet music with a 3X telescope and cap focused for 16 inches, what telescope and cap are needed to read the same sheet music set at 32 inches?

Magnification

23. A +40.00 D hand magnifier is used to view text placed 25 cm from the patient's eyes. Assuming the text is located at the focal point of the magnifier, what is (a) the angular magnification of the lens, (b) the effective magnification of the lens, and (c) the conventional magnification of the lens?

24. A +24.00 D lens is used as a handheld magnifier, with the patient viewing an object that is 50 cm away from the eye (and at the focal point of the lens). How much larger do things appear to the patient?

25. A patient says that her magnifier makes things 50 cm away look 4X larger. You rate the magnifier at 2X, but the box says that the power is 3X. You know that the manufacturer of this lens uses conventional magnification when labeling its products. What is the power of this lens?

CCTV

26. A patient can read newsprint on a CCTV through a standard add of +3.00 D, sitting approximately 13 inches from the screen. When measured, a 1 mm space on a ruler placed on the newspaper measures 12 mm on the screen. What lens would this patient theoretically need to read the same newspaper?

Field of View

27. What is the linear field of view of a 50 mm round +12.00 D handheld magnifier held 20 cm from the eye? Assume the object is at the focal point of the magnifier. What is the field if the magnifier is held 10 cm from the eye?

Answers

1. (a) +5 D (b) +7.50 D (c) +10 D (d) +15 D
2. 10 D
3. +10.00 D
4. (a) 20 D (b) 20 D
5. (a) +10.00 D (b) +6.00 D
6. +8.00 D
7. +14.50 D
8. +14.50 D
9. (a) +20.00 D (b) +10.00 D (c) 5 cm ($z = f_1$)
10. (a) with DV Rx (b) with DV Rx (c) with add
11. (a) 6X (b) +21 D
12. + 4.00 D add; 5 cm between glasses and stand magnifier
13. approximately 18 cm; 10.00 D
14. 20 cm; 2.5X
15. +10 D objective; −30 D ocular
16. 2X, 18.8 mm; 1.5X, 20.8 mm; 2.5X, 17.5 mm
17. 21.8 D
18. (a) 2X (b) 2.5 cm (c) 3.1 cm
19. (a) 29 D (b) +4.00 D
20. 2.5X telescope with a +4.00 D reading cap
21. 10 D
22. 6× telescope with +1.25 D cap
23. (a) 10X (b) 10X (c) 11X
24. 12 times
25. 8 D
26. +36 D add
27. 20.8 mm; 41.6 mm

7

Prescribing Conventional Lenses for the Low Vision Patient

Alan L. Innes

Key Terms

spectacles	lens thickness	aberrations
lens materials	lens tints	ptosis crutch
base curve	lens coatings	

Low vision patients most often seek care because they are having difficulty with near tasks. It is no surprise, therefore, that the focus of most low vision evaluations is on prescribing devices to improve the patient's ability to accomplish up close tasks. With the emphasis on near testing, the impact of the distance prescription on the function and well-being of the patient can easily be overlooked. This chapter will address the role of the distance spectacles in low vision therapy and then proceed to background and application of the lens materials, designs, and surface treatments. Fitting considerations, including measurements and frame selection, will also be discussed. The chapter will conclude with a discussion of the criteria for fitting and the fabrication of a ptosis crutch on a frame.

The goal of this discussion is to review and update the design and fitting of conventional spectacles which will enhance the utilization of the other devices that are prescribed, as well as being useful as a stand-alone item.

Prescription Considerations

Material Factors

There are several reasons to recommend a conventional pair of glasses for the low vision patient. The importance of the distance prescription from a clinical perspective, aside from an improvement in acuity, is that it will provide the baseline for low vision devices. From the patient's perspective, however, other aspects such as appearance may be at least as important as acuity.

CLINICAL PEARL

The importance of the distance prescription from a clinical perspective, aside from an improvement in acuity, is that it will provide the baseline for low vision devices.

There are cases which may warrant an alteration in the design of the patient's spectacles. For example, if the patient who has been wearing a flat top bifocal with a low add for reading experiences a significant decrease in acuity, the add power required to allow the patient to read the same size print may necessitate a switch to a kryptok in order to incorporate the new add. There may also be a need to make a change to a different material, or a lenticular from a full field. In some cases a spectacle-mounted telescope will require the fabrication of a whole new pair of spectacles even though no change in prescription is found. They may also be prescribed simply to protect the seeing eye in a monocular patient.

Patient Factors

There are also obstacles that may preclude the acceptance of distance spectacles. Frequently, low vision patients claim that their spectacles do them no good. If, however, they are tested on a chart at 10 feet or allowed to view a familiar object, with and without the spectacles, they will frequently observe clarity of the image with their spectacles.[1] In some cases the spectacles do not provide the patient with the desired acuity level. It may, however, still be prudent to provide the patient with distance spectacles since they do play a role in giving the patient a connection with the "real world" as compared to the nature of the visual handicap and the devices used for improved visual performance.

Regardless of the motivation for the low vision examination, conventional spectacles should be given the same consideration as any other aspects of the therapy since they are often an integral part of achieving the patient's goals.

Ophthalmic Materials

A large percentage of low vision patients have extraordinary prescriptions. High myopia, hyperopia, and astigmatism are common in this population. Special materials and lens forms will be utilized more often, on a proportional basis, for the low vision patient than in the normally sighted population.

Statistically speaking there are 11 different materials to choose from. They are, in order of index:

1. CR-39
2. Crown
3. CR-39 1.54
4. CR-39 1.56
5. CR-39 1.57
6. CR-39 1.58
7. Polycarbonate 1.586
8. CR-39 1.60
9. CR-39 1.66
10. Hilite 1.70
11. Index 8 1.81

Characteristics

With such a broad range of materials it should be easy to satisfy the criteria for optimum lens performance for most patients. Considering the profile of the individual we are usually working with, ideally the lenses should optimize optics for best visual acuity, strength for protection (especially in the monocular patient), and visible light transmission for contrast. Other important factors include UV absorption and weight. There is one other factor which also deserves our attention. A majority of the low vision population are elderly and will likely have problems with manipulative skills. When combined with their poor vision there is the strong possibility that spectacles will be mishandled or misplaced. Therefore the lenses should be durable enough to withstand a certain amount of abuse and mishandling. They should also be cost effective since there is the likelihood that the spectacles may be lost. This is an important consideration for many patients who are on a fixed income or depend on third party programs to subsidize their care. The choice, in some cases, will depend on what the patient is able to afford.

The optical and physical characteristics vary with index. As index increases, optics and durability are compromised and cost goes up dramatically. While there are several factors that can be used to guide the selection, the choice of lens material and design will often be based on the prescription. That will also dictate other features such as the frame characteristics, design, and centering, which will be discussed later in this chapter.

Optical and Mechanical Considerations

Most of the problems associated with strong lenses are greater for convex than for concave lenses.[2] Hyperopia presents a special problem in that the center of the lenses can be very thick, which (along with steeper base curves), plays a major role in the generation of magnification in a plus lens. According to the approximation

$$M(\%) = (t/n)F_1 + F_{BV}(V)$$

if we assume that the spectacles are fitted for minimum vertex distance, then the power factor (second term on right side of equation) remains constant. This implies that the shape factor (first term on the right), which is a function of thickness and base curve, will determine the magnification characteristics of the lens.

Magnification can affect the patient's visual performance in prescriptions over +5.00 D. The end result, particularly in aphakia, is that patients have to reorient themselves because objects appear larger and closer than they really are. The disorientation makes it difficult to walk around in unfamiliar surroundings. Even simple tasks such as pouring coffee can be a frustrating experience.[3]

In an aphake, the disparity can be as much as 25%. An object that is 8 feet away appears to the patient to be 6 feet away. Problems with high plus can also manifest, somewhat more subtly but equally as disturbing, in the form of a peripheral blind spot (ring scotoma) caused by the prismatic effect at the edge of the lens. As the back vertex power of the lens increases, the size of the scotoma increases.[4] High plus lenses also produce pincushion distortion which aphakic patients, in particular, will notice when wearing a spectacle correction.

The moderate to high myope presents a different set of problems which relate largely to appearance.[5] This includes not only the actual thickness, which can be quite objectionable, but also the minification effects which result in the appearance (through the spectacles), of the face being compressed. High minus lenses are heavier than plus lenses [6] and they generate considerable reflections from the surfaces because of the very flat and steep curvatures inherent in these lenses. From a clinical point of view, the practitioner also has an interest in controlling edge thickness to help reduce aberrations and maintain optical quality and cosmetic appeal.

Prescribing Basic Lens Materials

Although there is no single material which will optimize lens performance, CR-39 is considered to be the best all-around material for ophthalmic lenses. The fact that it is formulated with a low index of refraction makes this possible. It combines light weight with excellent optics, transmission, and durability. It is also relatively inexpensive when compared with high index materials. It is ideal for low power minus prescriptions and many plus prescriptions.

CLINICAL PEARL

CR-39 is considered to be the best all-around material for ophthalmic lenses.

Limitations

For all of its excellent qualities, however, CR-39 may not be the best choice for patients who require high prescriptions. In these prescriptions, CR-39 lenses will be thicker than lenses made with any other material and, when compared with high index plastic, they will also be heavier. This is manifested quite dramatically when CR-39 is used for high minus prescriptions. Depending on the eye size and the thickness of the semifinished blank, it may be impossible to achieve a full field design in a –15.00 D. If a full field lens is made, the edges may be so thick that they will touch the patient's face or, at the very least, not allow the temples to be folded. However, it is important to remember that the prescription may not be as useful to the low vision patient if the optical quality is sacrificed. For that reason CR-39 may often be the material of choice.

Utilization

In moderate to high plus powers, on the other hand, CR-39 is probably the best material to prescribe. It has excellent optics in that it is relatively free of chromatic aberration. Contributing to the superior optics is the fact that it is available on aspheric base curves. Since optics are of considerably more importance in plus than minus, it makes good sense to use a material which, above all else, provides good optics in the way of reduced chromatic aberration and surface accuracy. We also know that CR-39 is more dimensionally stable than other resin materials. This means that there is less of a chance that CR-39 will warp when subjected to heat and pressure. Both are important factors in the surfacing of any lens. This also contributes to the better optical quality found in a CR-39 lens.

Alternatives

There are several alternatives to CR-39 in fabricating high minus lenses. Even though high index may compromise acuity, it is the material of choice for high minus prescriptions because it is capable of providing lenses that are significantly thinner and lighter in weight. High index lenses are also manufactured with thinner than normal centers and, in some cases, aspheric base curves (in minus the inside curve is aspheric). What is sacrificed is optics. In most high index lenses, chromatic aberration is more likely to be a problem. They are also softer than standard materials and thus more prone to scratching, even with S/R coatings.

In minus lenses, thickness can be controlled by selecting a high index material. The higher the index the thinner the lens, all other parameters being equal. The idea behind the use of high index materials is that these materials require flatter curves to generate the same refractive power. According to the following relationship, flatter curves mean less thickness at the edge (Figure 7-1).

For example, if one were to order a −12.00 D lens, 60 mm in diameter, plano base curve, and 2 mm center thickness, the radius of curvature for the back surface would be 40.8 mm for a CR-39 lens and 58.3 mm for Hilite. That is, it would take a radius of almost 41 mm to generate the same power in CR-39 that could be achieved in Hilite with a radius of 58 mm. That represents a significant difference in surface radius which translates into a noticeable difference in edge thickness. Further calculation shows that the edge thickness would range from 14.8 mm on a CR-39 lens to 10.3 mm for Hilite. This represents a 30% difference in thickness. In between these two materials would be 1.6 index plastic at 12 mm, polycarbonate at 12.3 mm and crown at 13.7 mm.

Radius of curvature relative to index for 3 commonly used materials

$$F = -15.00 \qquad \text{Where } r = \frac{n' - n}{F}$$

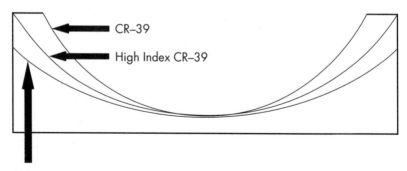

FIGURE 7-1 Diagram of minus lens showing how an increase in index generates a flatter surface leading to a thinner lens.

As (n′) increases, the numerator of the equation in Figure 7-1 increases with a resultant increase in the radius of the surface. A longer radius translates into a shallower surface.

If thickness and weight are the overriding concerns, one of the high index plastic lenses should be given consideration. The two high index materials used most commonly at the present time are high index CR-39, index 1.60; and polycarbonate, index 1.586. Both materials will provide about 15% to 20% decrease in edge thickness depending on the power and the minimum blank size. Both offer good impact resistance. However, polycarbonate is far superior in impact resistance to index 1.60 or any other material. Patients frequently complain about chromatic aberration and distortion with these lenses. CR-39, index 1.60 provides better optics and more scratch resistance. It is not as strong as polycarbonate, however. Both have limited application because they are not ordinarily available in prescriptions above −14.00 in the strongest meridian. In plus, both are available in powers up to about +8.00.

If all of these criteria are secondary to thickness considerations, Hilite or Index 8 (both titanium oxide based materials), are the materials of choice. Because Hilite has a very high index (1.70) the resulting lens will have an edge that is about 25% to 30% thinner than CR-39 or Crown and is treated by ion exchange to render it about as strong as a CR-39 lens. Although it is heavier per unit of volume than Crown, Hilite provides a large enough savings in thickness that it produces a lens, in prescriptions over −7.00 diopters, that is lighter than Crown in the same prescription and lens size. Being a glass material, Hilite is more scratch resistant than plastic. Even though Hilite has the same Nu value (30) as polycarbonate, the effects of dispersion seem to be less noticeable in Hilite than polycarbonate.

Consequences for the patient

What does this mean for the low vision patient? One aspect of vision that is often a problem is contrast. This is a function of clarity and illumination. Assuming that the spectacle prescription is optimum for the viewing distance, illumination is the only variable that can be altered. High index lenses reduce the amount of light available to the eye according to the following equation:

$$\text{Ref} = \left[\frac{n' - n}{n' + n}\right]^2$$

From the perspective of contrast, high index lenses may not be the best choice. In CR-39 the loss of light due to reflections is about 8%. In high index CR-39 the loss of light is about 10% to 12%. In the worst case scenario, the loss would be between 14% and 15%. The resulting reflections can be very problematic as it relates to the patient's vision. Again, this relates to the trade-off in physical versus optical performance.

> **CLINICAL PEARL**
>
> *High index lenses reduce the amount of light available to the eye according to the following equation:*
>
> $$Ref = \left[\frac{n' - n}{n' + n}\right]^2$$
>
> *Strictly from the perspective of contrast, high index lenses may not be the best choice.*

Lens Design

In spite of the large number of options available, lens materials alone cannot take care of all the problems that might arise when prescribing for low vision patients. The design of the lens may have to be altered to help in the overall performance or appearance of high power lenses or to overcome mechanical problems in the fabrication of a given pair of spectacles. This means that an existing lens may have to be modified or a special lens form may have to be ordered. There are some new designs such as low plus aspheric lenses and the Myothin process and minus aspherics, which have been introduced recently. All have had a significant impact on the hyperopic and myopic population in terms of optical performance and cosmetic enhancement.

Designs for Enhancing Optics

Modern corrected curve lenses are based on calculations that allow for the correction of marginal astigmatism and power error over a range of powers from about +8.00 to −24.00 D.[2] Most minus powers fall well within that range. We can see, however, that in prescriptions over about +8.00, marginal astigmatism and power error cannot be properly controlled by spherical corrected curve lens designs. This is why for the last three decades, all high plus (and now low plus) have been manufactured with aspheric curves on the front surface. This feature is also found on polycarbonate, and high index CR-39. This feature produces a lens that is not only optically superior to spherical designs, but also is better looking.

Aspheric lenses are a necessity for most hyperopic patients. They are now available for all hyperopic prescriptions (including the AO microscopic line of aspheric lenticulars which goes up to 12X). The primary advantage of aspherics is that flatter curves can be used while maintaining a lens that is relatively free of aberrations. This type of design is particularly useful for controlling distortion, which can be a major adaptation stumbling block.

CLINICAL PEARL

The primary advantage of aspherics is that flatter curves can be used while maintaining a lens that is relatively free of aberrations.

As a general rule, no matter what the material or prescription, all lenses, whether single vision or multifocal, should be ordered as full field whenever possible. When a full field lens is not practical from a mechanical point of view, the alternative is a lenticular lens form. Either of these can be designed as meniscus, biconcave, or biconvex, depending on the prescription. Meniscus lenses are always the most desirable because they provide the best optical qualities. It is helpful to avoid flat surfaces since they can emphasize reflections. The box on p. 184 provides a representative, but not necessarily comprehensive, listing of designs available without special order.

CLINICAL PEARL

As a general rule, no matter what the material or prescription, all lenses, whether single vision or multifocal, should be ordered as full field whenever possible.

CLINICAL PEARL

Meniscus lenses are always the most desirable because they provide the best optical qualities when compared with other forms.

Single Vision vs. Multifocals

If a patient needs both distance and near prescriptions, the least complicated solution from a mechanical perspective is a separate set of distance and reading glasses. This offers the advantage of minimizing the possible confusion which arises for some patients when trying to move around with bifocals on. For those patients who require a strong add, the blur through the segment when trying to look at their feet can temper enthusiasm for wearing a bifocal. The disadvantage lies more in the fact that the patient has to keep track of an additional pair of glasses.

Multifocals

A majority of the patients examined in low vision practice can achieve improved reading performance if given a higher add. For many of

---

⬤Plus Aspheric Lens Design

Variable aspheric: full field only
Low to medium powers (+0.25 to +12.00)
   Base curve varies according to lens power by 0.25 to 2.00 diopters.
   Several brands available in CR-39, 1.54, polycarbonate, and 1.60.
High powers (+10.00 to +20.00)
   Fulvue aspheric
   Super modular aspheric
      On both designs the base curve varies between 2.50 to 5.00 diopters
      depending on lens power.
Fixed: high powers only
   Aspheric lenticular
      2.50 diopters of power change on base curve
      40 mm optic zone
      *Also available in prefabricated microscope form in powers up to 12X
   Full field
      4.00 diopters of power change on base curve
        Multi-drop
          Also with prism segment in flat top
        Hyperaspheric

All designs available in single vision or in flat top and, in lenticular, a round segment.

---

these patients the additional plus can be used effectively in the form of a bifocal. This type of correction offers two advantages over single vision spectacles.

1. It eliminates the need to carry two pairs of spectacles.
2. It is cosmetically more appealing.

Frequently the add power prescribed will be higher than that given a normally sighted patient. In very high adds or situations that call for unusual prescription components such as prism, there may be a question about the availability of a bifocal to fit the prescription parameters. Except in very rare instances there is always a lens, either stock semi-finished or custom made, which will fill the requirements.

All conventional bifocals are available in stock semifinished form with add powers up to +4.00 D. Many are made with adds as high as +6.00. There are at least three designs—flat top, round seg, and Ultex A—made by several companies, with adds as high as +10.00. Add powers up to +20.00 can be ordered in plastic round segment bifocals and Ultex A.

When ordering add powers over +5.00 or +6.00 D it is advisable to do a monocular fitting unless the patient can alternate easily from one eye to the other. It is difficult for the patient to use higher adds binocularly because of the close working distance. If the patient prefers to have a binocular correction and the distance prescription is negligible, the prefabricated half eye or full field prism spectacles are the best choice or a lens can be made to incorporate base in prism in the segment to reduce convergence demand (Ben Franklin Multifocals, to be discussed later in the chapter). If the patient cannot wear a bifocal due to personal choice or because of poor mobility, the alternative would be prefabricated aspheric lenticular which, again, can only be fit monocularly.

Fitting

The important parameter in the fitting of the high add patient is the segment height. High add bifocals should be fit higher than the standard segment height (to the lower lid). There are two reasons for fitting these lenses this way. First, with the segment higher, the patient will be able to get into the useful part of the segment with a minimum of downgaze. This also means that there will be less prismatic effect vertically because the visual axis will be closer to the distance optical center. The second reason is that it will usually allow the patient to see under the segment. This is helpful for going up and down steps or simply when walking about outdoors.

CLINICAL PEARL

The important parameter in the fitting of the high add patient is the segment height. With the segment higher, the patient will be able to get into the useful part of the segment with a minimum of downgaze. It will usually allow the patient to see under the segment.

For any bifocal (and high adds in particular), modifying the inset relative to the working distance is usually not crucial since the fitting is done monocularly. Under this condition the patient will turn the head to align the segment with the visual axis. If the patient does not respond well to this posture, a considerable amount of inset can be incorporated into a round segment bifocal. The same cannot be accomplished with a straight top segment.

The patient should also be fit with an adjustable bridge frame so that minor adjustments can be made should the patient require a change in the positioning of the segment.[7] In some cases it may be helpful to fit the Focal Change Frame. This is a relatively new design incorporating an adjustable bridge that slides up and down on tracks on either side of the bridge. This allows the patient to have the pads up, in normal position (Figure 7-2), or move the bifocal up higher by moving the pads down (Figure 7-3) when doing close work. This has

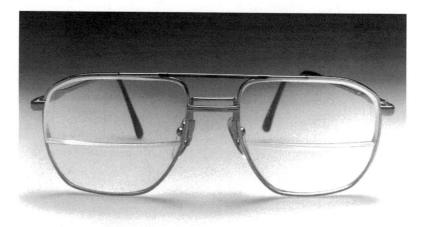

FIGURE 7-2   Focal Change Frame: normal position, pads up.

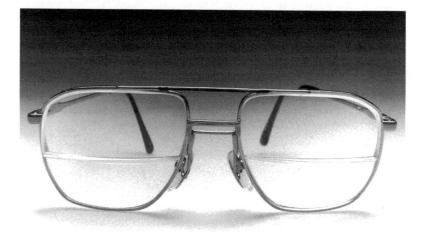

FIGURE 7-3   Focal Change Frame: bifocal is higher with the pads shifted down for close work.

the obvious advantage of allowing the patient to adjust the position of the segment depending on the task at hand.

Ben Franklin Multifocals

As mentioned earlier, there will be situations in which a conventional bifocal will not fulfill the prescription requirements. For example, this could be a case where prism is required at distance or near, but not both; or a high add with a large field of view.

The answer to this problem is to design an executive style bifocal from two single vision lenses or, in the case of a trifocal, fabricated from an executive bifocal and a single vision lens. These are called (for obvious reasons) Ben Franklin Multifocals. They offer greater flexibility with regard to segment height, add power, prism at distance or near, intermediate powers, and intermediate width. (See Figures 7-4, 7-5, and 7-6.)

The height measurement for this type of lens is usually the same as for a standard executive.

Fitting Considerations

As with other devices the patient will be using, the spectacle correction in a new material or design may require some adaptation time. This can also happen, of course, when there are significant prescription changes. Therefore it is of considerable importance that the spectacles be fit with due consideration for the frame size, base curve, and frame adjustment. This will help keep adaptation time to a minimum.

Base curve has already been discussed as it relates to spherical versus aspheric configuration. Although minus lenses are available with aspheric curves on the inside of the lens, it is in plus prescriptions that aspherics are most useful. Otherwise spherical surfaces will

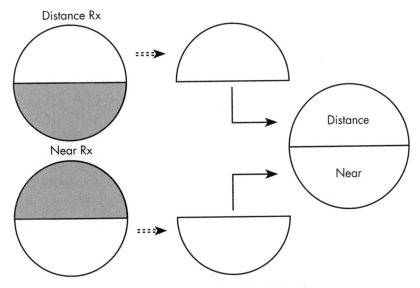

FIGURE 7-4 Ben Franklin Bifocal

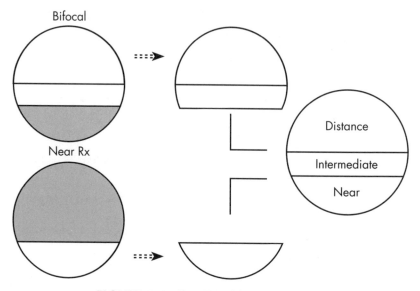

FIGURE 7-5 Ben Franklin Trifocal

suffice. In higher powered prescriptions, there is little opportunity to manipulate the surface powers because specific curves must be used. It is impractical to specify a base curve in most cases.

The frame is an important consideration in helping the low vision patient to realize the full potential of a pair of spectacles. Selecting a small frame with a symmetrical shape can make a significant contribution to controlling edge and center thickness, and to reducing the compressive effects of minus lenses and magnification effects in plus. The frame should fit as close as possible and be the same width as the patient's head. It should have enough bulk to create a balanced pair of spectacles. This will also help cover the edges of the lens.

Careful measurements will also help improve the chances that the patient will adapt to their lenses. For moderate to high prescriptions monocular Pds taken with a pupillometer are essential. This will also reveal any asymmetry in the patient's Pd as well as give an accurate measurement. It is also usually necessary to take a vertical height measurement, as is done in progressive lens fitting, to get the optical centers in alignment with the patient's visual axes in their habitual viewing posture. This measurement is usually taken to a point midway between the lower lid and lower pupil border (mid-iris).

Lens Enhancements

Although the use of high index materials can contribute significantly to the appearance of a high minus lens, there are other things that can be added to the basic lens to help in this regard. The first thing that can

Bifocal   Trifocal

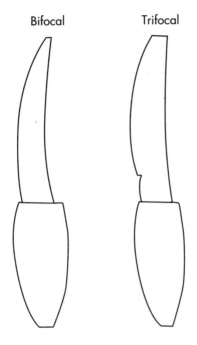

FIGURE 7-6 Profiles of the Ben Franklin Bifocal and Trifocal.

be done is to add an antireflection coating. In fact, this is something which should be added to all high minus lenses.[4] The coating should be a double-sided multilayer (usually 5 or 6 layers on each side). This will reduce the intensity of reflections. Other useful surface treatments are tinting (which should be about the same color as the frame), edge polishing, and edge coating.

To protect the patient, other lens treatments such as ultraviolet coatings and tints are often useful. UV 400 coatings offer aphakes and patients with macular disease, protection from all ultraviolet radiation. This feature will help minimize the possibility of further damage to an already compromised eye.

Filters

Although symptoms and eye conditions can predict the type of filter the patient will wear, ultimately it is the patient's subjective response that will guide the decision on which filter to wear. Filters are prescribed to protect the patient from the harmful effects of ultraviolet or infrared radiation and to reduce the amount of visible light getting to the eye, to help the patient with general light sensitivity. Filters can also be prescribed to help improve contrast.

The decision about how to provide a filter for the low vision patient depends on the prescription, cost, and the patient's preference. Since most of the filtering lenses provided today are either dyed or coated, the decision depends less on the prescription than it did in the past. If a composition type of tint (absorptive properties manufactured in lens material through the addition of the appropriate oxide) such as Calobar, Cosmetan, or True Color is considered, the prescription is the most important consideration. Lenses made by this method should not be used in prescriptions above + or – 4.00 D because of the density differences that result from significant thickness differences inherent in higher powers. In powers over 4.00 D, coated glass, dyed plastic, clip-on, or NOIR or UV Shield should be used.

The ideal vehicle for providing filters for the low vision patient is a separate pair of spectacles with the desired tint. Patients requiring several devices to satisfy their needs may opt for a fit-over or clip-on to help contain the cost of the devices. A word of caution should be noted here about the use of polycarbonate. The structure of polycarbonate does not allow it to be tinted to densities greater than about 55% or 60% even with the tintable scratch coating. When polycarbonate is used, clip-on filters can be worn over tinted polycarbonate lenses if the density of the dye does not provide enough protection. Clip-on filters, however, should be used with caution because the clips or the lenses in the clip-ons can scratch the polycarbonate lenses.

Photochromic lenses have been in existence for many years. They are available in brown and grey in a wide variety of lens types. There is also a plastic version available. They, like the glass photochromic lenses, are temperature sensitive but considerably more so. In warm weather they do not darken very much outdoors. In cold weather they get darker than glass photochromics; in many cases too dark for a majority of patients. They are essentially fashion tints with little applicability for low vision patients.

Corning's well-known CPF series has proven to be of some help to low vision patients on a limited basis. They are fabricated in densities with transmissions starting at 450 nm, 511 nm, 527 nm, and 550 nm. They are available in single vision and a limited range multifocal. Younger Optics has a series of single density (nonphotochromatic) plastic lenses in flip-up form with densities of 530, 540, and 550. They are similar in color and absorptive characteristics to the Corning lenses but, as noted previously, are not photochromatic.

Filters can also be supplied in the form of clip-on plastic sheets that slide behind the patient's spectacles (Instant Sunwear), or as prefabricated filters by NOIR and Solar Shield that can be used over the patient's habitually worn spectacles or by themselves. They come in grey, grey-green, amber, green, yellow, orange, plum, and red. Most are available in transmissions ranging from 1% to 65%. All of the Noir, Solar Shield, and UV Shield filters are UVA and short blue protective.

Polarized lenses are available in a greater variety of forms than at any time in the past. They are available in glass and plastic in single vision and multifocal as well as clip-ons and photochromatic. They are considerably more expensive than any of the other filters with the possible exception of the Corning CPF series. Clip-ons are the least expensive way to provide polarized filters to the patient.

Ptosis Crutch

Ptosis is a common ocular consequence of diseases like myasthenia gravis. It also presents as a congenital problem. Although it can be treated by surgery, this is often an unsuccessful approach. Patients with ptosis can be helped by mechanically elevating the lid with a double-sided tape made specifically for this purpose. Although effective, it is difficult to manipulate and costly.

A more practical approach is to employ a crutch device that can be attached to the patient's spectacles. The keys to the success of a ptosis crutch are the frame, the type of wire used, and the structure of the lid. The frame should be thick enough where the eyewire and bridge connect, so that a 0.22 inch diameter hole can be drilled with a #74 drill bit. The 0.22 gauge wire is fed through the hole(s) and given a slight bend to lock the wire in place so it cannot back out. The wire goes back to the superior sulcus by the trochlear notch, is then bent to conform to the superior sulcus, and places enough pressure on the lid to hold it in the desired position. The wire is then cut so that the end is just short of the temporal canthus. The end of the wire is bent out and up, and a piece of silicone tubing (like that found in the butterfly kits used to do the injection in fluorescein angiography) is used to cover the wire. This will make the crutch more comfortable and provide the eye protection from injury by the wire. To avoid pressure on the eye by the crutch, the wire must be bent to conform to the curvature of the eye with a slight push up toward the brow bone.

Most patients can achieve satisfactory visual and cosmetic results with a ptosis crutch. An elevation of 2 to 3 mm is sufficient to provide both. Success can often be predicted through the history and an appraisal of the superior lid structure. Those who have not had lid surgery and who have normal lid structure (a tarsal fold and a normal superior sulcus) will usually be successful. If the patient is proptotic the contour of the lid is such that it is difficult to position the crutch so that it will hold the lid in an elevated position.

References

1. Faye EE: *Clinical low vision*, ed 2, Boston, 1984, Little, Brown & Co, 27-44.
2. Morgan MW: High powered lenses. In Morgan MW: *Optics of ophthalmic lenses*, Chicago, 1978, Professional Press, 309-327.
3. Dowaliby M: *The art of eyewear dispensing*, ed 1, Fullerton, Calif, 1987, Southern California College of Optometry, 26-29.

4. Fannin TE, Grosvenor T: *Clinical Optics*, ed 1, Chicago, 1987, Professional Press, 359-389.
5. *The handbook of plastic optics*, ed 2, Cincinnati, 1983, US Precision Lens, Inc, 17-29.
6. Wohlover D: *Dispensing the latest ophthalmic lens products*, Minneapolis, 1990, Walman Optical Co.
7. Mischen C: Principles in fitting glasses. In Faye EE (ed): *Clinical low vision*, Boston, 1984, Little Brown & Co, 161-167.

For more information

Allergan Humphrey. Frames Product Guide. Lenses Supplement, December 1989;26;21.
Bonsett-Veal JD: Enhancing the cosmetic appearance of high minus spectacle lenses, *Optom Month* 12-23, January 1984.
Dowaliby M: *Practical aspects of ophthalmic optics,* ed 2, Chicago, 1980, Professional Press, 157-163.
Musikant S: Optical materials: an introduction to selection and application, Pioli, Pa, 1985, Marcel Dekker, Inc, 23-58.
Pentax Opthalmic Inc, Technical information monograph, Minnetonka, Minn, 1989, 1-9.
Pitt DG: Ultraviolet absorption by spectacle lenses, contact lenses, and intraocular lenses, *Optom Vis Sci* 67:435-440, 1990.

C H A P T E R

8

Visual Function with High-Tech Low Vision Devices

Gregory L. Goodrich
Theresa Sacco

Key Terms

add-on board	GUI (graphical user	personal computer
Americans with	interface)	reasonable
Disabilities Act	hardware	accommodation
application	icon	reading machine
program	large print access	scanner
computer access	program	software
copy protection	operating system	voice synthesizer

High-tech low vision aids provide clinicians an array of tools of unprecedented power in maximizing the functional vision of patients with severe visual impairments. The success of these devices is attributable to their inherent benefits and to changes in the U.S. educational, vocational, and social climate. In this chapter we will discuss the emergence of these devices, explore the importance of incorporating them into clinical practice, and provide clinical guidelines useful in prescribing them.

The Emergence of High-Tech Low Vision Aids

As early as 1959 the potential use of video technology in low vision was discussed by Potts and his colleagues.[1] As great as this potential was, the creation of a commercial product required another decade before closed-circuit televisions (CCTVs) emerged as commercially viable products. The first CCTVs were large, expensive, and cumbersome devices which, while generally well received, stimulated some controversy.[2] Subsequent improvements in these devices coupled with price reductions spurred their acceptance so that by the end of the decade they were widely accepted as the preeminent low vision aid for reading tasks.

At the same time that CCTVs were being accepted in low vision clinics, major innovations were being made in computer technology. Two of these innovations, speech technology and the development of the microprocessor chip, would have profound effects upon vision rehabilitation. By the early 1980s the first personal computers (such as those made by Apple, Osborn, Kaypro, and others) were introduced to the world. Initially these inexpensive computers were greeted with a good deal of skepticism by computer specialists who had only experienced mainframe computers. The first Apple II computers, for example, seemed extremely limited (having less memory than current electronic appointment calendars), yet the rapid evolution of the microprocessor chip allowed personal computers to rapidly become a significant force in schools and the workplace.

As quickly as the Apple II computer invaded classrooms, special education teachers and others began to add the newly developed speech technology to these computers so that visually impaired students could share in learning to use these exciting new tools. By the late 1970s and early 1980s it seemed that between reading machines and computers, the print barrier separating blind and sighted individuals would be torn down. Voice output terminals and personal computers led to major improvements in education and helped promote the concept of mainstreaming blind children. Microprocessor technology also allowed text enlargement so that personal computers could be used by partially-sighted individuals with large print and/or speech. This same technology potentially opened many new occupations to people who were visually impaired and today there are individuals in professions ranging from engineering to the law—thanks to the development of the microprocessor. Unfortunately, while many individuals who are visually impaired have benefited from the new technology, not all barriers have been overcome and the potential for most remains a potential, not a reality.

Society's stereotype of "the blind" remains a barrier. The Americans with Disabilities Act and other legislation have chipped large holes in the walls separating visually impaired individuals from the workplace, but individuals who are blind or partially sighted remain among the most underemployed and unemployed of all minorities.

The very pace at which microprocessor technology has advanced has also become a barrier. Computer operating systems are "improved" two or three times a year, and a truism of application software is that if you can purchase it, it is already obsolete and the "new" version will be on store shelves within a few months. This rapid pace of change has made it difficult for those writing access software and creating access hardware to stay current with the latest technology.

CLINICAL PEARL

Computer operating systems are "improved" two or three times a year, and a truism of application software is that if you can purchase it, it is already obsolete and the "new" version will be on store shelves within a few months.

The recent proliferation of graphical user interfaces (GUIs) is an apt illustration. The translation of text into speech is a relatively straightforward undertaking; word groupings are simply "read" by the computer. GUIs, however, use symbols (icons) and spatial position to encode information, and it is difficult to translate such complex information into usable speech. GUIs present less of a problem for large print access since they can easily be enlarged by many large print access programs. Still they are not without problems. The enlargement of a portion of the computer monitor results in a small portion of the screen being visible at any given moment. In effect the access program creates an artificial "tunnel vision" with which the user must cope, as well as coping with the visual impairment.

CLINICAL PEARL

The enlargement of a portion of the computer monitor results in a small portion of the screen being visible at any given moment. In effect the access program creates an artificial "tunnel vision" with which the user must cope, as well as coping with the visual impairment.

These and related difficulties challenge the partially-sighted computer user and the clinician who seeks to prescribe high-tech low vision devices. Any technical solution to large print computer access tends to be transient in its effectiveness. It is almost as if the computer software companies are continually striving to make any access solution obsolete. The clinician and the partially-sighted computer user may feel they are in a situation in which they must constantly learn new skills just to maintain a constant level of access to computers.

In the past several years the number of large print software application programs has grown dramatically,[3] and a resource guide to the majority of Macintosh- and IBM-compatible programs is contained in the spring issue of the *Aids and Appliances Review*.[4] This is an extremely helpful guide for the clinician prescribing high-tech devices since it provides a description of the features of each product and contact information for the manufacturer. Clinicians are well advised to contact each manufacturer and ask to be placed on its mailing list, which will allow them to become aware of new or modified products.

Access to computers by visually impaired individuals does not always require a high-tech device, nor is visual access always the optimum means of accessing a computer. According to the National Eye Institute[5] (1994) most of the 3 million individuals in the United States with impaired vision are classified as severely visually impaired. In general terms one can consider these individuals to have visual acuities of between 20/50 and 20/200 and/or visual fields of not less than 40 degrees. About 900,000 of these 3 million people are classified as sighted, but legally blind. That is, they will have usable vision, but best corrected visual acuities of 20/200 or less and/or a visual field of 20 degrees or less. Blind individuals, with light perception or less, number about 100,000 individuals.

CLINICAL PEARL

Access to computers by visually impaired individuals does not always require a high-tech device, nor is visual access always the optimum means of accessing a computer.

Experience has shown that computer users in each of these three groups can benefit from different types of computer access devices. The three types of access are: (1) conventional low vision (near) devices, (2) large print computer access programs, and (3) voice or braille computer access.

Conventional Low Vision Devices

The majority of visually impaired individuals who work with computers can benefit from such conventional low vision aids as high plus lenses, bioptics, clip-ons, and others (Figure 8-1). The range of visual acuities for which this is true does not have a hard-and-fast definition.

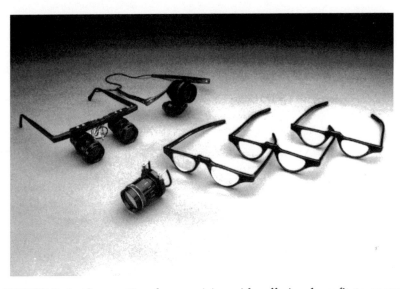

FIGURE 8-1 Conventional near vision aids offering benefit to some visually impaired computer users.

In general, however, optical aids become less effective (in comparison to large print access programs) as visual acuity decreases. McGillivray has found that most patients with visual acuities of 20/200 or less will benefit less from optical aids and more from large print software.[6] Our clinical experience tends to confirm this; however, there can be a substantial gray area such that clinicians may want to evaluate patients with acuities above and below this cutoff for both optical aids and large print access programs.

CLINICAL PEARL

Patients with visual acuities of 20/200 or less will benefit less from optical aids and more from large print software.

In addition to optical aids, substantial benefits can be derived from simple and inexpensive modifications to the work environment and the computer. Among these are the following:

- The low vision computer user (like any low vision patient) will benefit from learning about, and how to control, lighting, glare, and other environmental illumination problems. This can include the use of Fresnel prisms which reduce glare and reportedly reduce visual fatigue for many people. Fresnel prisms that can be attached to computer monitors are readily available in computer stores and through catalogue sales.

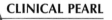

CLINICAL PEARL

The low vision computer user (like any low vision patient) will benefit from learning about, and how to control, lighting, glare, and other environmental illumination problems.

- Monitor stands can be used to comfortably position the monitor and take advantage of approach magnification. Increasing the monitor size from 13 inches to 25 inches also provides an image that is about 2X larger, although the cost is also significantly greater for the larger monitor (Figure 8-2).
- Computer monitors provide many of the same advantages as CCTVs. They provide high quality images, good contrast, and

CLINICAL PEARL

Computer monitors provide many of the same advantages as CCTVs. They provide high quality images, good contrast, and (usually) the ability to control color contrast.

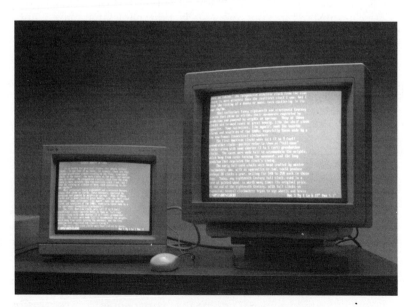

FIGURE 8-2 Magnification can be provided via a larger monitor, as well as via an access program.

(usually) the ability to control color contrast. The clinician needs to ensure that patients understand how to use these features of the computer monitor to maximize their visual performance.

Large Print Computer Access Programs

Once the use of optical aids has been ruled out, the next step is to consider large print access programs. These are software programs that enlarge the text, menus, graphics and/or icons displayed by the computer. As previously stated, clinical experience has shown that these programs are of most benefit to patients whose visual acuity is 20/200 or less. This holds true for patients with considerably less vision, up to those whose visual needs require magnification such that only five or six characters can be displayed at one time on the monitor. At this level the patient's reading performance is generally so slow as to warrant consideration of nonvisual access techniques. These will be discussed in the next section.

The number of large print access programs has grown, in the past few years, from a mere handful to some 30 different programs,[3,4] including the few shown in Figure 8-3. The rate at which new programs are introduced, and existing programs modified, makes it virtually impossible to write a current article on any single access program. Therefore we will address general features of interest and concern that the clinician can use in successfully working with the low vision computer user.

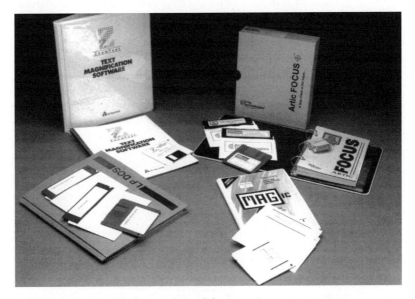

FIGURE 8-3 Software-based large print access programs.

Patient Sophistication and Computer Activities

The clinician working with large print access will find that his or her skills as a low vision clinician will be extremely useful, and that additional skills will need to be learned. For example, an important consideration is the level of computer sophistication of the patient. Those who are extremely proficient may need very little support beyond learning where to purchase the access program. At the other extreme, computer novices will benefit from a clinician who takes the time to understand their computer needs and who provides assistance in locating a computer access training facility. In this case the clinician and the computer access training staff can form a team to meet the patient's needs.

The novice computer user is likely to want a computer solely for word processing tasks or as an entry level tool for learning about computers. In such cases, one of several dedicated large print word processing programs (i.e., Flexiwrite from Laird Communications in Manchester, Massachusetts) is easily learned and used for word processing. The computer sophisticate would likely benefit from an access program that provided access to various applications such as word processing, databases, spreadsheets, graphics, terminal emulation programs, and others. These programs, while versatile, can be challenging even to the computer sophisticate and consideration should be given to enrolling in a computer access training program.

Large Print Access from PCs to Mainframes

Some large print access products support stand-alone PC use, and also support linking a PC to networks and mainframe computers. When using a PC to emulate a terminal (for example, when connecting to a mainframe), it is important to consider that the transfer of commands/information from the PC to the mainframe (and back) will require frequent updates of the monitor display. Some large print access programs will not be able to cope with these updates, and the PC-to-mainframe connection will fail. A general rule of thumb to follow is that a large print access program that uses an add-on board should be used in these situations (Fig. 17-4). These boards provide extra memory and minimize the problems encountered in connecting personal computers to mainframes due to frequent screen updates.

Computer Sharing and Transportability

Computer users often need to work with computers in more than one location, and they may need to share their computer with sighted colleagues. These considerations may restrict the number of access programs that are viable for the individual. If the computer is to be shared, the patient will want to ensure that the visual display can easily shift between magnified and normal views. If computers at more than one location are used, either the access program has to be duplicated at each computer or it must be transported. This is not possible for some programs which employ copy protection schemes limiting the number of times the master program can be installed, and the prudent clinician and patient will check with the manufacturer to learn whether this is the case or not. Other access programs require the installation of an add-on board, as well as software installation (Figure 8-4). These are not easily transported; therefore a purely software-based access program is preferred.

Hardware Requirements

Many access programs have specific hardware requirements. That is, they will only work with certain types of equipment. Some, for example, work only with VGA compatible monitors while others work with CGA and EGA monitors. To make matters worse, some manufacturers make video adapter cards which may not be compatible with the access program even if the monitor is. A simple rule of thumb minimizes these problems: Try out any access program on the computer system it is to be used with before it is purchased. This will save time and money, and reduce both the clinician's and patient's frustration.

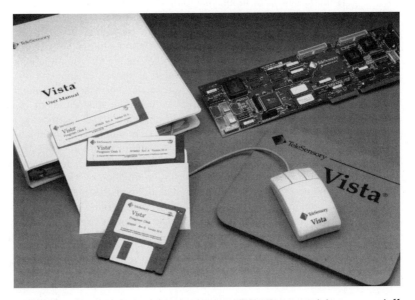

FIGURE 8-4 Vista, a large print access program requiring a specially built add-on board, and controlled via a mouse.

CLINICAL PEARL

Try out any access program on the computer system it is to be used with before it is purchased. This will save time and money, and reduce both the clinician's and patient's frustration.

Access Control and Other Features

Computers have traditionally been controlled by commands entered on the keyboard, but the more recent GUIs require the use of a mouse or sometimes a joystick. Access programs are also controlled via the keyboard, and some are controlled by a mouse. It is possible that conflicts can occur between the GUI operating system, the application program, and large print access program. That is, two (or more) of these may use the same command for two different tasks. In such cases the result is that the computer freezes or "crashes." Again, the rule of thumb of trying it out before purchase will minimize these problems.

GUI Large Print Access Considerations

The basic set of instructions that govern the functions of a computer is called its operating system. The operating system controls all aspects of the computer from input, manipulation, and display to storage on disk. The earliest personal computers used text-based operating systems that required the user to enter alphanumeric text to get the computer to perform a function. Such text-based systems, although less flashy than more recent operating systems, had a distinct advantage for visually impaired users in that text could easily be converted to speech or enlarged text. The more sophisticated GUI operating systems (i.e., the Macintosh operating system, Windows, and OS/2) perform very similar functions; but in addition to using text, they require the user to point a cursor (by moving a mouse) to particular spatial locations on the monitor. The information at such locations may be in the form of an icon (or picture) or it may be in the form of a pull-down menu. Once the icon or menu is selected with the mouse and cursor, the user can activate the function by clicking a button on the mouse. The use of icons significantly increases the difficulty of creating a computer that is fully accessible to a totally blind individual. It also creates new concerns for partially-sighted computer users. The following points are relevant when prescribing large print access for computers that employ GUI operating systems:

- Not all large print access programs support GUIs. Check with the manufacturer before purchase.

- There are differing levels of sophistication between GUI (and DOS) access programs. Some offer limited features at the GUI level, while others offer extensive features allowing the user to optimize the display to his or her own visual characteristics.
- Even if the access program supports GUIs there may be other equipment incompatibilities. (Please note: some manuals refer to "appropriate" hardware without defining the term.) Check with the manufacturer to ensure that the access program contains appropriate printer, monitor, and video drivers.
- The fonts and quality of characters supported by different access programs vary. Some display smoothly formed characters on the monitor, while others support only stair-stepped or jagged characters. For many partially-sighted individuals, there is little visual difference between smooth and jagged; however, it is best to ensure this before purchase.
- Access programs vary in their scanning speeds. Some scan at rates too high for many partially-sighted users, thus it is necessary to ensure that the access program scanning speed can be adjusted. Also, in some access programs the scan rate can only be adjusted in some viewing modes (e.g., fully magnified) and the user should determine if such limitations would hinder computer use.
- The readability of GUI displays can be enhanced (for some users) by changing background and foreground colors, but not all access programs support this function. It may be very helpful for your patient if you ensure that the program supports color monitors.
- When using an access program with a GUI operating system, the mouse takes on extra functions. A priority conflict can occur when the access program, operating system, and/or application program calls for a given mouse action to do different tasks. Such conflicts (if they exist) usually become obvious only when the access program is used in real world tasks. For this (and other reasons) it is advantageous to try out the access program prior to purchase.
- In selecting between GUI access programs it is important to ensure that the access program easily switches between levels of magnification and from magnified to unmagnified views.

There are also other considerations that characterize any good DOS or GUI access program and work environment, and the conscientious clinician will review these with the patient. Consideration should be given to the patient's vision and the work environment. For example, the computer monitor should be able to tilt for comfortable viewing and the room lighting should be adequate for reading, but with no glare sources. The patient will also benefit from an understanding of how to manipulate the contrast and brightness features of the computer, and how to change the display font to one that is easily read. A near correction should be explored for the working distances used at the computer, and presbyopes should be prescribed an appropriate near add. The computer desk and chair should have good ergonomic characteristics, and a reading stand for print materials and references can be beneficial.

Other features that should be considered are: How easy to read is the access program's manual? Can it be understood by a novice or does it require an expert? Does the access program provide a sufficient and comfortable range of magnifications? Can the user preprogram (and store in memory) the preferred access configuration so that the computer does not have to be "set up" each time it is used?

The low vision clinician will likely find that his or her patients are interested in computer access, and following the above guidelines will assist in meeting these patients' needs. One spur to this increased interest has been passage of the Americans with Disabilities Act which mandates that reasonable accommodation must be provided. Reasonable accommodation has, in many instances, been interpreted to mean that if a student or employee is provided a computer, a visually impaired person in the same position must also be provided an accessible computer. As a result many schools and universities have started computer access programs, and businesses are increasingly purchasing the needed access equipment and providing the training needed by their visually impaired employees. The costs involved are indeed reasonable, ranging from a few hundred dollars to several thousand dollars. Even at the high end of this range the cost is reasonable both in terms of the cost of any computer equipment and the cost of keeping a worker productive.

Alternatives to Visual Access

Some low vision patients will have visual requirements for magnification that are prohibitive. Our experience has been that in cases where the needed magnification limits the number of characters on the screen to six or fewer, voice or braille computer displays may be more efficient. The low vision clinician should be aware of these alternatives and be prepared to recommend them should the patient's visual performance warrant it. For some patients a combination of large print access and nonvisual access will be beneficial. Among the nonvisual options that can be considered are stand-alone reading machines that provide access to printed material (Figure 8-5) and computer systems with scanners that convert text to digital signals and voice output (Figure 8-6). Patients can often find assistance in learning to use these devices through local agencies for the blind, junior college and university disabled student services, and/or state departments of rehabilitation.

CLINICAL PEARL

Our experience has been that in cases where the needed magnification limits the number of characters on the screen to six or fewer, voice or braille computer displays may be more efficient.

CLINICAL PEARL

For some patients a combination of large print access and nonvisual access will be beneficial.

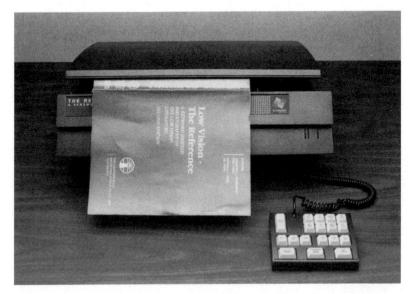

FIGURE 8-5 The Reading Edge. A stand-alone reading machine.

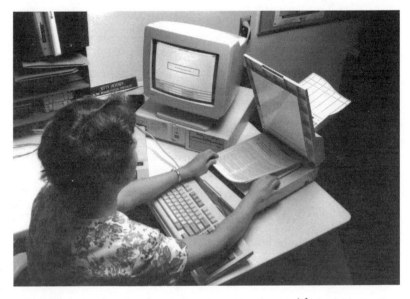

FIGURE 8-6 A voice input computer system with text scanner.

Summary

Since the early 1970s technology has produced remarkable aids for partially-sighted individuals. The CCTVs pioneered by Dr. Sam Gensensky provided remarkable access to printed materials.[7] The more recent development of personal computers has also created new opportunities for many individuals with low vision. Access to computers can be gained by conventional optical aids and by specialized large print access programs. For patients with extremely reduced visual function, computers can be accessed through a combination of large print and voice or braille output. Large print computers represent a new area for the clinician to expand the low vision practice and to provide an educationally and vocationally satisfying service to many patients.

CLINICAL PEARL

Access to computers can be gained by conventional optical aids and by specialized large print access programs. For patients with extremely reduced visual function, computers can be accessed through a combination of large print and voice or braille output.

References

1. Potts AM, Volk D, West SW: A television reader as a subnormal reading aid, *Am J Ophthalmol* 47:580-581, 1959.
2. Freidman GH: The closed circuit television reading system: fact or fiasco? *New Outlook for the Blind* 67:346-351, 1973.
3. Goodrich GL, Krueger N, McKinley JL: Large print computer access: 1993 options, *J Vis Rehabil* 7:20-24, 1993.
4. Author: Resource guide, *Aids and Appliances Review* 15:23-51, 1994.
5. Low Vision and Its Rehabilitation Panel: Report of the Low Vision and Its Rehabilitation Panel. In National Advisory Eye Council, National Eye Institute, *Vision research: a national plan 1994-1998*, Bethesda, Md, 1994.
6. McGillivray R: Comprehensive computer access evaluation for persons with low vision, *Aids and Appliances Review* 15:2-8, 1994.
7. Genensky SM, Baran P, Moshin HL, et al: A closed-circuit TV system for the visually handicapped, *American Foundation for the Blind Research Bulletin* 19:191, 1969.

C H A P T E R

9

Clinical Strategies for the Visually Impaired Computer User

John E. Musick

Key Terms

computers	components of	ergonomic
VDT screens	magnification	telemicroscope
source documents	equivalent viewing	
keyboard	distance	

Increasing numbers of the visually impaired population today desire to have access to and use computers, both at work and at home. This is due to the increased utilization of computers in society for a vast number of tasks as well as technological innovations that make it possible for the visually impaired to have access to computers. Consequently eye care practitioners are increasingly faced with the challenge of determining how patients with vision impairments can achieve and maintain access to computers most efficiently and cost effectively. This chapter deals with clinical considerations and strategies useful in helping patients with low vision to achieve their goals.

Functional Case History Considerations

Obtaining a detailed case history will greatly assist the clinician in deciding which clinical test procedures to perform as well as beginning to formulate appropriate management strategies. The general ophthalmic case history will usually include demographic information, the chief complaint, secondary concerns, and patient and familial ocular, visual, and general health history. When evaluating and managing low vision patients, it is especially necessary to determine their vision-related goals and desires as specifically as possible. This information will be useful in allowing the clinician to determine which specific optical and nonoptical options, if any, are most likely to enable patients to achieve their goals. For low vision patients who use (or desire to use) computers, gaining a better understanding of any previous computer experience as well as future anticipated computer use will help the clinician to develop a rationale for testing and managing patients. A sample questionnaire is given in this chapter. From patient information gained from these questions, additional interviewing can be conducted as the clinical evaluation proceeds. The case history will help to clarify the specific types of tasks the computer will be used for. Computer tasks may be classified in a variety of ways. The low vision clinician is primarily concerned with what percentage of time the patient spends viewing the video display terminal (VDT) monitor—also called the computer display screen—in comparison to the source documents (copy) and keyboard (keytops) or other objects in the computer work station environment. Activities such as data entry are very document intensive and indicate that the user spends the vast majority of time viewing the documents or printed data that must be entered into the computer.[1] Tasks such as data acquisition or computer programming may be very screen intensive with practically all of the time being used to view the VDT screen and only rarely viewing documents or the keyboard.[1] Other tasks such as word processing or interactive types of computer activities will find the user varying the amount of time spent between viewing the screen and documents. Understanding the patient's vision-related computer tasks and their relative importance to each other will greatly assist the clinician in planning appropriate clinical management strategies.

CLINICAL PEARL

The case history will help to clarify the specific types of tasks the computer will be used for.

CLINICAL PEARL

Activities such as data entry are very document intensive and indicate that the user spends the vast majority of time viewing the documents or printed data that must be entered into the computer. Tasks such as data acquisition or computer programming may be very screen intensive with practically all of the time being used to view the VDT screen and only rarely viewing documents or the keyboard. Other tasks such as word processing or interactive types of computer activities will find the user varying the amount of time spent between viewing the screen and documents.

In summary, the low vision clinician utilizes the case history to gain sufficient information to help determine the patient's potential to use remaining vision to accomplish one or more of the tasks necessary to use the computer satisfactorily. These vision-related tasks include viewing one or more of the following objects: the VDT screen, the source documents, and the keyboard.

Among the most useful clinically available strategies for improving visibility and resolution of these objects is altering the retinal image size of one or more of the objects by changing one or more of the components of magnification that determine the retinal image size of the objects.

CLINICAL PEARL

Among the most useful clinically available strategies for improving visibility and resolution of these objects is altering the retinal image size of one or more of the objects by changing one or more of the components of magnification that determine the retinal image size of the objects.

For many patients, there are several possible options that could be made clinically that will result in a change in retinal image size. The clinician has the responsibility to first evaluate the magnification requirements (i.e., needed changes in retinal image size) for each task at the computer work station. These determinations can be made in a variety of ways and one relatively quick and reliable method is based upon determining the equivalent viewing distance (EVD)[2] for each task. The EVD is the distance that the original object (i.e., the VDT screen characters, documents/copy text, or keyboard keytops) would have to be positioned in order to be satisfactorily seen or read with only a conventional spectacle lens worn to correct for a refractive error and accommodative demands. It is equivalent to utilizing only relative

A Sample Case History Questionnaire for Vision Impaired Computer Users

Experience

Have you had any previous experience using computers? If so, for what task or activities did you use computers? For what types of tasks do you anticipate using computers in the future? What portion of your time at work, home, or school will you likely be using computers?

Training

What formal computer training, if any, have you already obtained? Do you plan to take any formal computer training in the future? If so, when and where will you obtain this?

Hardware and software

What types of computer hardware and software have you previously used or are you familiar with? What types of hardware or software do you anticipate using in the future?

Effect of vision impairment on computer use

How does your vision affect your use of computers? What changes, if any, have occurred in your vision since you first began to use computers? Has this change in vision caused difficulty with any tasks associated with computer use? If so, what (if anything) has been done to help compensate for this change?

Typing/keyboard skills

What typing skills, if any, do you presently have? Are you thoroughly familiar with the computer keyboard? Will you need to have any formal training in keyboard or typing skills to enable you to accomplish your present and future computer tasks?

Ergonomic considerations

Have you experienced any discomfort, pain, or dysfunction in your body or your eyes while working with computers? If so, please specify. Do any of these problems still exist? What (if anything) was done to relieve them?

Utilization of lenses and nonoptical devices

Do you wear glasses or contacts or use any optical or nonoptical devices when using the computer? If so, which glasses/contacts or devices and for what specific task? Do you use any special software or hardware to help compensate for your vision impairment? If so, please specify.

distance magnification (M_{dist}) to provide the total magnification needed to satisfactorily view the object/task at its original size. The EVD is usually expressed in centimeters and when expressed in diopters (100/EVD in centimeters) is called the equivalent viewing

The Components of Magnification

Relative distance (M_{dist}) - Changing the viewing distance of an object causes an inversely proportional change in the retinal image size of the object.

Relative size (M_{size}) - Changing the actual size of the object being viewed will cause a directly proportional change in retinal image size, assuming no change in viewing distance.

Angular (M_{ang}) - Changing the apparent size of the object through the use of a telescopic lens system will cause a change in retinal image size proportional to the magnification (X) strength of the telescope.

Display ($M_{display}$) - Changing the size of an object displayed on a VDT or TV screen through special computer software/hardware or CCTV will cause a proportional change in the retinal image size.

Total magnification (M_{total}) obtained is equal to the product of each of the individual components of magnification:

$$M_{total} = M_{dist} \times M_{size} \times M_{ang} \times M_{display}$$

power (EVP).[2] Once the needed EVD (or EVP) is reliably determined for a specific task, changes in one or more of the clinical options for each task can be considered as long as the total magnification will be at least equal to the needed EVD/EVP for that particular task.

The VDT Screen

The VDT viewing screen or video monitor display is the object most unique to the computer user with respect to most other traditional work-related equipment. The visual display of a VDT can be generated by either a cathode-ray tube (CRT) or as a liquid crystal display (LCD)[3] and in many cases rivals the quality of printed text. The advantages to the visually impaired user are the options to easily change display character size, contrast, color, and character design. The disadvantages include limitations on the physical placement of the VDT screen in the computer work station and undesirable reflections of surrounding sources of illumination off the display screen. Possible solutions to reducing the reflections off the display screen include first identifying them by placing a mirror over the screen to directly visualize and determine the origin of the glare sources. Management options include repositioning the VDT monitor or the glare sources. Alternately, modification of existing fluorescent lighting fixtures through the use of a parabolic fixture or louver (parawedge) beneath the fixture will help minimize the horizontal dispersion of light. The use of micromesh or polarizing antiglare screens may also help to diminish bothersome reflections.[4]

Determining the EVD/EVP for Computer Tasks

Step 1:

Determine the size of the characters or text that must be seen for each computer related task. This is most accurately determined by actual analysis or examination of the various tasks/objects or can be approximated as follows:

VDT display characters (alphanumerics): 10 point (1.2M) and larger.
Documents/copy (text):   Typed print = 12 point (1.5M)
                          Newsprint = 8 point (1.0M)
Keyboard (keytops):   Letters = 18 point (2.2M)
                          Numbers/symbols = 14 point (1.7M)

Step 2

Determine the farthest distance from the patient's eyes that the patient can read/see the task with acceptable accuracy and efficiency. Try to use the actual task/objects, if available clinically, to make this determination. Be sure to provide lens corrections appropriate for the patient's refractive error and the test viewing distance to ensure that the retinal image is in acceptable focus. Note the effects of varying the illumination and whether the patient performs better monocularly or binocularly.

Step 3

Record the distance found in step 2 for each task and the size/characteristics of the test/objects used. This distance now becomes the equivalent viewing distance (EVD) for that particular task.

Example

You determine that the farthest distance a low vision patient can comfortably read VDT screen characters (12 point) is 20 cm. She can also see her reference documents (8 point) at 13 cm and keytops (14 point) at 25 cm.

For this patient, the respective EVD/EVP are as follows:

12 point VDT characters: 20 cm/5 D
8 point documents (newsprint)   13 cm/7.75 D
14 point keyboard (keytops)   25 cm/4 D

CLINICAL PEARL

Possible solutions to reducing the reflections off the display screen include first identifying them by placing a mirror over the screen to directly visualize and determine the origin of the glare sources. Management options include repositioning the VDT monitor or the glare sources. The use of micromesh or polarizing antiglare screens may also help to diminish bothersome reflections.

The VDT display characters are made up of individual dots called pixels. The resolution of the monitor is often defined by the number of rows and columns of pixels on the screen. Higher numbers for the same size screens indicate more densely spaced pixels resulting in higher resolution and better legibility. Another factor influencing VDT display character resolution is the dot pitch, a measure of the spacing between the VDT screen's individual phosphors. The smaller the dot pitch, the sharper the display characters appear.

Options for the VDT Screen

Options for altering the retinal image size of the VDT screen characters/figures are listed in Table 9-1. The clinician must consider both the optical and functional consequences of each possible option as it relates to the user's clinical findings and case history. Moving the VDT monitor significantly closer may require utilization of additional office equipment such as a support stand with a counterbalanced arm appropriate for the monitor size and weight. If the user will have to look back and forth from documents/copy to the VDT screen, greater

TABLE 9-1

VDT Options

Clinical strategy	Type of magnification	Example
Change the distance between the VDT screen	M_{dist}	Moving a VDT from 60 cm to 30 cm will provide 60/30 or 2X enlargement.
Switch to a different size monitor	M_{size}	Switching from a 12 inch screen size to a 21 inch screen will provide a 21/12 or 1.75X increase in size.
Using a bioptic telemicroscope to view the VDT screen	M_{ang}	Viewing the screen through a 3.0X near vision telescope will provide a 3X enlargement.
Using a large Fresnel-type magnifier in front of the VDT screen	M_{ang}/M_{dist}	These work like very large but low-powered stand magnifiers. A +3D diopter lens positioned 15 cm in front of a VDT screen (which itself is located 50 cm from the user) will only provide a 1.5X enlargement.
Using special software programs to display enlarged figures on the screen	$M_{display}$	A software program that enlarges the characters by factor of 8 will provide an 8X enlargement.

head and eye movements may be required and could result in ergonomically unacceptable changes in the user's posture. Lens corrections of appropriate power and design will need to be considered based on changes in viewing distances and the task positions of all objects that need to be seen by the user at the work station. Using software with enlarged size display characters will cause a proportionate decrease in the number of characters that can be displayed at any one time.

CLINICAL PEARL

Moving the VDT monitor significantly closer may require utilization of additional office equipment such as a support stand with a counterbalanced arm appropriate for the monitor size and weight.

CLINICAL PEARL

Lens corrections of appropriate power and design will need to be considered based on changes in viewing distances and the task positions of all objects that need to be seen by the user at the work station.

Options for Viewing the Documents/Copy

Options for altering the retinal image size of the documents or copy that the user is required to see while working at the computer are listed in Table 9-2. Moving the copy closer will usually require the use of an adjustable copy stand and consideration similar to moving the VDT closer. If the copy has to be frequently changed, excessively close copy distances may necessitate awkward or uncomfortable hand/arm movements and body postural changes that will be detrimental from an ergonomic standpoint if user task time is lengthy. Adequate lighting must be provided to view the copy but positioned so that it does not create undesirable glare off the VDT screen and into the user's eyes.

CLINICAL PEARL

If the copy has to be frequently changed, excessively close copy distances may necessitate awkward or uncomfortable hand/arm movements and body postural changes that will be detrimental from an ergonomic standpoint if user task time is lengthy.

TABLE 9-2
Documents/Copy Options

Clinical strategy	Type of magnification	Example
Change the distance between the user and the documents	M_{dist}	Moving the copy from 50 cm to 20 cm will provide 50/20 or 2.5X enlargement.
Recopy the documents to enlarge them	M_{size}	Recopying the copy on a setting of 150% will make the characters 1.5X larger.
Use a bioptic telescope to view the copy	M_{ang}	To determine the required magnification of a telescope, divide the desired viewing distance (e.g., 50 cm) by the needed equivalent viewing distance (e.g., 20 cm) 50/20 = 2.5X.
Use a CCTV camera to project an enlarged image of the copy onto a separate TV monitor or VDT screen itself	$M_{display}$	If copy that is actually 8 point in size is projected to appear 40 point in size, 5X enlargement is attained.

Using a copy machine to enlarge the copy can be relatively costly and inefficient both in terms of time and reproduction expense. If a CCTV is used to enlarge the copy, a movable x-y table with a motorized foot control may be more efficient and comfortable than continually changing the position of the copy beneath the CCTV camera manually.

Bioptic Telemicroscopes

A telemicroscope system, if utilized, would generally be used to view both the copy and the VDT screen since it potentially becomes an undesirable object in the patient's field of view when it is not being used. A telemicroscope, when compared to a spectacle add or microscope of the same equivalent power, has a longer viewing distance by a factor equivalent to the magnification of the telescope. However, the depth of field (region where the object will remain in acceptable focus when the viewing distance is changed) is no greater than the equivalently powered microscope or reading add.[5] Thus if a telemicroscope is used to view both documents and copy, care must be taken to place each at essentially the same viewing distance and as close to each other as possible to avoid having to refocus the telemicroscope and to minimize the amount of head movement needed to change fixation from one task to the other. The linear field of view of a telemicroscope (expressed in centimeters) is equal to its angular view (expressed in degrees) when objects are viewed through the telescope at 57 cm. Thus a telemicroscope with a 12 degree angular field has a linear field of view of 12 cm when used to view objects located 57 cm away. To determine the approximate linear field of view (in centimeters) of a telescope used to view at a specific near distance, multiply the angular field of view (in degrees) by the ratio of the viewing distance (in centimeters) divided by 57 cm. Thus a 3.0X telemicroscope with an angular field of view of 10 degrees, when used to view at 40 cm, will have a linear field of view of 10 × 40/57 or 7 cm.

CLINICAL PEARL

A telemicroscope, when compared to a spectacle add or microscope of the same equivalent power, has a longer viewing distance by a factor equivalent to the magnification of the telescope.

CLINICAL PEARL

If a telemicroscope is used to view both documents and copy, care must be taken to place each at essentially the same viewing distance and as close to each other as possible to avoid having to refocus the telemicroscope and to minimize the amount of head movement needed to change fixation from one task to the other.

To determine what magnification strength to choose initially when using a telemicroscope, multiply the total EVP needed to perform the task (see box on page 214) by the desired viewing distance expressed in meters. For example, assume that a patient requires a total EVP of +12 diopters in order to read his copy when working at the computer. If the copy is placed at 25 cm (0.25) he would require a telescope magnification of +12 diopters × .25 or 3X. If the patient decides to position the copy further away, say at 33 cm, the needed magnification strength of the telemicroscope would be +12 diopters × .33 or 4X. The linear depth of field will actually be the same for each telemicroscope system that has the same total equivalent power (magnification strength of telescope multiplied by the viewing distance expressed in diopters).[5] Thus while the actual viewing distance is increased, the depth of field remains the same linearly. If the 3X and 4X telemicroscopes had exactly the same angular field of view, the 4X system would have a greater linear field of view at the greater viewing distance by an amount equal to the ratio of the 4X telescope's viewing distance divided by the 3X telescope's viewing distance. Clinically, a higher powered telescope usually will have an inherently smaller angular field of view than a lower powered telescope and, frequently, there is no real increase in the linear field of view when using a greater viewing distance.

Options for the Keyboard

There are not as many practical options for viewing the keyboard as compared to the VDT screen or copy. Serious computer users generally become thoroughly familiar with the position and location of the 100+ keys on the computer keyboard. Having or acquiring excellent-typing skills is especially advantageous for the visually impaired since such skills will almost eliminate the need for the user to have to view the keys and will lessen the number of typing (entry) mistakes. It is usually not ergonomically acceptable to change the position of the keyboard with respect to the optimal working position for most users. It is recommended that the user's elbows are bent approximately 90 degrees, the forearms are supported by armrests, and the wrists and hands are extended nearly straight to the keyboard.[6] Perhaps the most satisfactory and effective means to improve visibility without creating undesirable consequences is to use keytops with enlarged characters. These are relatively inexpensive and provide slightly more than a two-fold (2X) increase in size magnification. They are available in standard contrast (black characters on white keytops) or reverse contrast (white characters on black keytops). Some VDT monitors with touch sensitive screens may allow for the keyboard to be displayed and operated by physically touching the screen with the user's fingers or remotely by use of a mouse or other device.

CLINICAL PEARL

Keytops with enlarged characters are relatively inexpensive and provide slightly more than a twofold (2×) increase in size magnification.

What are the Practical Limits on Magnification?

The clinician is faced with the reality and challenge of having to recommend clinical strategies for computer users with a wide range of functional vision requirements, clinical findings, and differences in functional visual capabilities. In some cases, it will become readily apparent that using vision as the primary modality to carry out one or more of the computer tasks may not be possible or the most efficient means. Clinically there are practical limits on magnification that should be kept in mind. For instance, if the user decides to rely primarily on relative distance magnification (M_{dist}) to improve VDT screen characters or copy, viewing distances much closer than about 4 cm are usually unacceptable. This is due to the short depth of field and the need to make head and eye movements of rather large magnitudes in order to see various regions of the screen or copy. This is especially significant when both screen and copy must be alternately seen. This would mean a practical limit of 4 cm/25 D for the EVD/EVP obtainable through M_{dist}. If such a patient could read 12 point (1.5M) text at 4 cm, this would imply that the patient's functional reading capabilities would need to be approximately 120 point (15M) at 40 cm. This would correlate roughly with a functional distance Snellen equivalent of 20/750.

When considering relative size magnification (M_{size}), the average VDT diagonal screen size currently used is about 14 inches and the largest VDT diagonal screen size currently available is about 27 inches. Thus based on a VDT viewing distance of 50 cm, the practical limit of magnification based solely on changing the size of the monitor is 27/14 or about 2X. The EVD/EVP would be 50 cm ÷ 2 or 25 cm/4 D. For angular magnification (M_{ang}) the strongest bioptic telemicroscope system clinically useful is about 6X due to the short depth of field and narrow field of view. If a 6X telemicroscope with an angular field of view of 6 degrees is used to view text at 24 cm, the linear field of view at 24 cm is only 2.5 cm wide. The total EVD/EVP for this system is 4 cm/25 D. This narrow field of view will also limit using additional components of magnification such as display magnification ($M_{display}$) since it will further limit the number of characters that can be seen through the telescope at any one time. When considering $M_{display}$, there are currently several software programs that will provide up to 12X enlargement (with the highest being 16X) of the VDT screen characters or graphics. Assuming a reference distance of 50 cm for viewing the screen, the EVD/EVP for a $M_{display}$ of 12X would be 50 cm ÷ 12 or about 4 cm/24 D.

> **CLINICAL PEARL**
> *The largest VDT diagonal screen size currently available is about 27 inches.*

Considering Nonvisual Options

The actual clinical testing and evaluation with low vision devices and computer work station equipment usually helps the clinician decide which system or combination of systems may be most effective and useful for a particular patient. Part of this evaluation should include a determination of the user's efficiency at performing the task for those clinical strategies that are being considered. If it is determined that the task cannot be completed at a satisfactory rate or not at all using vision based strategies, nonvision based methods of accomplishing the task must be considered. The eye care practitioner may wish to consult with an assistive technology specialist to help determine which nonvision based strategies would be most appropriate. It is helpful to provide results and impressions from the vision based evaluation that the practitioner has conducted and indicate which strategies seem most feasible. In some instances, a patient may use two sensory modalities to perform one or more tasks at the computer work station. This will be especially important if reduced visual functions significantly slow information processing or increase time required to complete certain tasks. For example, if the user is employing vision based strategies to read text on a VDT screen and can only read a maximum of 60 words per minute (wpm), using a speech output device and listening to the text being spoken may increase the work rate. Typical speech rates are usually between 100 and 200 wpm and certain listeners can process up to 300 wpm. However, when the information content is very high, the user will have to slow the listening rate or resume using a vision based modality such as large display software.

CLINICAL PEARL

Typical speech rates are usually between 100 and 200 wpm and certain listeners can process up to 300 wpm.

References

1. Grandjean E: Ergonomics for VDUs: review of present knowledge. In Grandjean E, Vigliani E (eds): *Ergonomic aspects of visual display terminals,* London, 1983, Taylor and Francis Ltd.
2. Bullimore MA, Bailey IL: Stand magnifiers: an evaluation of the new stand magnifiers from COIL, *Optom Vis Sci* 66(11):766-773, 1989.
3. Boyce PR: Lighting and lighting conditions. In Roufs JAJ: *Vision and visual dysfunction,* vol 15, *The man-machine interface,* New York, 1991, The Macmillan Press Ltd.
4. Sauter SL, Schnorr TM: Occupational health aspects of work with video display terminals. In Rom WN (ed): *Environmental and occupational medicine,* New York, 1992, Little, Brown & Co.
5. Spitzberg LA, Qi M: Depth of field of plus lenses and reading telescopes, *Optom Vis Sci* 71(2):115-119, 1994.
6. Hunting W et al: Constrained postures of VDU operators. In Grandjean E, Vigliani E (eds): *Ergonomic aspects of visual display terminals,* London, 1983, Taylor and Francis Ltd.

10

Low Vision Driving among Normally-Sighted Drivers

Kent E. Higgins

Key Terms

visual impairment	night driving	bioptic driving
low vision driving	visual acuity	civil twilight
vision standards for driver licensure	visual fields	elderly drivers

The publication of *Transportation in an Aging Society, Special Report 218*,[1,2] served to underscore the important role of the automobile and the driving privilege for maintaining the quality of life of the older individual. Employment, health care, and numerous everyday activities depend heavily on the individual mobility it provides. This same report also served to underscore the rapid changes in the age distribution of the population. In 1900, less than 5% of the American population was over the age of 65. By 1988, the number had grown to 12%. By the year 2020, the number is expected to reach 17%, with 50 million persons of this age eligible to drive.[3] This trend becomes particularly significant when viewed in the context of additional data indicating that, in terms of automotive crash risk, older drivers may constitute the most hazardous group of drivers in the population.[3]

> **CLINICAL PEARL**
> *Older drivers may constitute the most hazardous group of drivers in the population.*

There has, accordingly, been a greatly renewed interest in identifying the influence of various age related factors that might place the older driver at greater risk on the roadways. It is obvious that there can be nonvisual changes with age (e.g., dementia)[4] that are important for safe driving. However, this chapter will focus on the possible role of vision in driving. Age related declines in visual function have been well-documented.[5-7] One important implication of these changes is that an increasing number of the elderly can be expected to fail the prevalent visual standard for driver licensure, the acuity test. For purposes of licensure, they will be considered "low vision" individuals. In addition, it is worth recalling that over two thirds of all people with low vision are over 65 years of age.[8] Consequently the aging of the population will force licensing agencies to continue to evaluate the issue of the low vision driver and, importantly, the justifiability of their vision standards for licensure.

It is virtually impossible to read the literature on driving and vision without encountering a statement to the effect that 90% of the information required for driving is visual.[9,10] On this point, there would appear to be little argument. Unfortunately, no one has yet provided the empirical evidence that could be used to define exactly what that statement means. After several decades of research and speculation [11,12] on the role of vision and driving, we still have very little empirical evidence concerning the minimal visual requirements for driving.

> **CLINICAL PEARL**
> *To date, no convincing empirical evidence has shown that the increased risk of accident involvement in the elderly is due to losses in vision per se.*

Prevalent Vision Standards for Licensure

One seemingly obvious way to try to answer the question about the minimal visual requirements for driving would be to refer to state vision standards for driver licensure.[13,14] Currently, for example, all states screen new applicants for visual acuity, requiring (in most cases) an acuity of 20/40 or better in at least one eye for an unrestricted personal driver's license. In addition, roughly one third to one half of the states list a minimal horizontal visual field requirement. A few states also include a provision for testing such visual characteristics as color vision and depth perception. However, even fewer use the results of such tests as a basis for the denial of licensure.[15]

More importantly, surveys of state vision requirements for licensure provide a confusing picture of what the minimal visual requirements for driving might be. Close inspection of any of the several surveys of vision standards for driver licensure reveals that there are significant variations across states, even when one considers the most prevalent vision standards: visual acuity and visual fields. For example, some states provide those individuals who are not able to meet their vision standards for unrestricted licensure with an opportunity to obtain a special restricted driver's license (e.g., daytime-only driving) while others do not.[16,17] Variations in the vision standards for licensure reflect our current state of ignorance about the role of vision in driving.

CLINICAL PEARL

Variations in the vision standards for licensure reflect our current state of ignorance about the role of vision in driving.

Bioptic Driving: A Misplaced Focus?

In the past, most of the more vigorous debates concerning the visual requirements for driving focused on bioptic driving.[18-30] Should individuals be allowed to use a telescopic device (a bioptic) as an aid, both while taking the visual acuity test and while driving? In principle, the logic of this procedure is simple. Assume that a state requires 20/40 visual acuity in the better eye as a minimal visual requirement for licensure. An individual with 20/120 best-corrected spectacle acuity would, while viewing through a 3X bioptic, be able to read the 20/40 line on the visual acuity test chart and therefore satisfy this vision requirement.

However, there ensued a vigorous exchange of opinion concerning the use of the bioptic for the driving task. Opponents of bioptic driving claimed that the bioptic itself would represent a potential driving hazard. For example, it was argued that, when looking through the bioptic, the bioptic housing would create a "ring" scotoma.[23] Such a scotoma could interfere with the driver's field of view and might therefore offset any gain in visual acuity attributed to the use of the bioptic.

Proponents of bioptic driving, however, argued that this viewpoint represented a misunderstanding of how the telescope would be used for driving. They argued that the bioptic would typically be mounted in the upper half of one of the individual's spectacle lenses and would, in addition, be angled slightly upward. The spectacle lens, also known as the carrier lens, would contain the refractive correction providing the 20/120 level of acuity in this example. To view through the telescope, the individual would have to momentarily dip the head slightly and elevate his or her gaze. From this perspective, the bioptic driver's use of the telescope as a driving aid could be likened to the normally-sighted driver's use of a rear view mirror as a momentary "spotting" aid.[25]

This latter point is critically important for any discussion of the minimal visual requirements for driving. If, for the sake of argument, we assume that the bioptic would be used for only about 3 to 5 seconds per driving minute, it would mean that only 5% to 8% of total driving time would involve viewing through the bioptic. The remaining 95% to 98% of total driving time would have to be based on whatever vision could be supported by the carrier lens. In terms of the previous example, this would imply that our hypothetical bioptic driver would be driving with the 20/120 visual acuity and lateral field of view provided by the carrier lens. The important point of this oversimplified example is that it serves to refocus the discussion away from the subject of bioptic driving and toward the subject of carrier lens driving.

Accordingly the next section will review the more traditional research design that has been used to try to evaluate the role of vision in driving without bioptics. The objective of this section is to offer speculation about why so much research has accomplished so little in terms of clarifying our understanding of the visual requirements for driving. The final section will be devoted to the development of the hypothesis that the visual requirements for driving may be more modest than those implied by current vision standards for driver licensure. The impatient reader, wishing to anticipate the rationale of this latter point, can do so by considering the following question: If visually impaired individuals are to have their driving privileges restricted or denied, should not normally-sighted individuals have their privileges restricted or denied when their vision is similarly impaired?

Brief Review of Traditional Research on Vision and Driving

The model for most of the research attempting to define the role of vision for driving was set by the early pioneering work of Burg and collaborators.[31-33] Briefly the approach consisted of correlating measured visual characteristics thought to be important for driving with some measure of driver performance (typically traffic accident and/or traffic violation record). Burg's battery of vision tests included measurements of static and dynamic visual acuity, lateral visual field, lateral heterophoria, low-light recognition thresholds, glare recovery, and sighting dominance. Burg's study was conducted on 17,500 California drivers. Considering the magnitude of the study, the results must have been considered a disappointment. Correlations between vision tests and driving records were weak at best. Although there were some statistically significant correlations (e.g., static, acuity, dynamic acuity, and visual fields), the magnitude of all were less than 0.1. Since the proportion of variance accounted for is proportional to the square of the correlation coefficient,[34] it was clear that vision test results were of little value in predicting real world accidents. Thus although such correlations sometimes achieved statistical significance, they achieved little in the way of practical significance.

CLINICAL PEARL

Numerous studies have repeatedly shown that vision tests like visual acuity are, at best, only weakly predictive of accident involvement.

Since that time there have been numerous additional studies, all of which have used basically the same "mass-screening" approach in an attempt to predict driving performance from measures of visual performance.[35-44] All were similar insofar as they relied on either self-reported or state-recorded traffic accidents and/or violations as a measure of driver performance. The results of all of these studies were also similar. Vision tests were, at best, only weakly predictive of accident involvement.

There are a number of hypotheses that might explain why the statistical linkages between vision and accidents were so weak in these studies. According to one hypothesis, the "fault" lies with the visual measurement procedures. It can be paraphrased by saying that we are not measuring the right visual characteristics and/or we are measuring them the wrong way. This hypothesis is implicit in the succession of mass-screening studies that have been carried out since the original work of Burg. Subsequent studies differed primarily in terms of the particular psychophysical methods used to measure vision and/or the particular visual functions tested.[35-44] Thus the poor predictive power of vision tests was blamed either on the selection of inappropriate tests or inappropriate test procedures.

More recently a test of visual attention has been described which would appear to be more predictive of accident involvement. This test, called the Useful Field of View Test (UFOV) is described as a test of visual attention.[43,44] Briefly summarized, this test measures a subject's ability to correctly identify central field targets while simultaneously having to localize peripheral field targets, both in the absence and in the presence of distracting targets. For a sample of elderly drivers, a correlation of 0.52 between the results of this test and crash frequency was found. By comparison, more conventional measures of vision such as visual field and contrast sensitivity were much less predictive of accident involvement. The authors of the study concluded that their data implied that current visual screening techniques, such as tests of acuity and peripheral vision as used at driver licensing sites, are not adequate in identifying which elderly drivers are likely to be involved in crashes.[44] However, before concluding that vision testing for driver licensure should be abandoned, consider a second hypothesis.

This hypothesis states that the relevant visual characteristics were, in fact, measured in many of the mass-screening studies by Burg and his successors. According to this hypothesis, the failure of existing vision standards is more apparent than real. To understand this statement, it is necessary to consider the end result of implementing a vision standard for driving that was, in fact, valid. Assume that a visual acuity of 20/__ represents the minimal visual acuity necessary for safe (i.e., accident-free) driving. This standard, if implemented, should have the effect of eliminating any accidents that could be blamed on poor visual acuity. If this vision standard were supplemented by an additional and valid visual field standard, accidents due to visual field loss should also be eliminated. If current vision standards are so restrictive as to effectively eliminate accidents that could be blamed on deficient vision, the expected correlation between accidents and vision test results is zero.

CLINICAL PEARL

If current vision standards are so restrictive as to effectively eliminate accidents that could be blamed on deficient vision, the expected correlation between accidents and vision test results is zero.

In this case, it is unlikely that we would interpret the low correlation coefficients as indicating the inadequacy of existing vision screening tests. Rather we would be more likely to conclude that our vision standards were so successful (i.e., sufficiently restrictive) that we had effectively eliminated any accidents that could be explained by reference to deficient vision. The critical empirical question is, what is the value of 20/__? The most prevalent vision standard is 20/40. However, as Bailey and Sheedy[45] have noted, in the absence of evidence to show that any particular level of visual acuity is required for driving, the common standard of 20/40 has evolved by consensus.

Present vision standards for driver licensure appear to be based more on historical sanction than on scientific fact.

CLINICAL PEARL

Present vision standards for driver licensure appear to be based more on historical sanction than on scientific fact.

The important question for an increasingly older society to ask is, how many elderly and low vision drivers would benefit from the driving privilege if it could be shown empirically that, for example, 20/120 was sufficient visual acuity for safe driving? An answer to the numerical part of this question could, in principle, be estimated. Unfortunately, it would be difficult to obtain the necessary empirical evidence, given the current practice of screening out individuals with acuities less than 20/40.

Low Vision Driving by the Normally-Sighted

This final section will be devoted to the question posed earlier: If visually impaired individuals are to have their driving privileges restricted or denied, should not normally-sighted individuals have their privileges restricted or denied when their vision is similarly impaired? The impartial answer to this question would be yes, but that answer could result in significant restrictions on driving by the normally-sighted individual.

CLINICAL PEARL

The ability of the normal visual system to resolve fine spatial detail varies greatly with light level.

It is a well-known fact that the spatial and temporal resolving power of the human visual system decreases from daytime photopic light levels to nighttime light levels.[46-48] Leibowitz and Owens[49,50] have pointed out parallels between early astronomical distinctions and their own attempts to understand twilight and nighttime driving. Early astronomers, they noted, distinguished three phases of twilight associated with sunrise and sunset, each lasting about 30 minutes and each representing a solar transit of about 6 degrees. Of particular importance is the approximately 2 log unit (100-fold) change in ambient light level during the brightest phase, of civil twilight. In the evening, the beginning of civil twilight occurs when the upper edge of the sun is tangent with the horizon. The end of this period (about 30 minutes later) occurs when the center of the sun is approximately 6 degrees below the horizon. At the brightest phase of the civil twilight period, the level of ambient outdoor illumination supplied by the setting sun is sufficient to ensure that most visual functions, including visual acuity, are at their normally high daytime levels, levels akin to those that would be obtained at motor vehicle testing centers.

However, as Leibowitz and Owens[50] have noted, the 100-fold reduction in ambient light level that occurs from the brightest to the dimmest phase of evening (or morning) civil twilight begins a rapid and selective decline in certain visual functions. Early astronomers regarded the decline as sufficient to suggest that normal outdoor activities could not be carried out with light levels less than the dimmest phase of civil twilight. Visual acuity is one such function that begins a rapid decline from the beginning to the end of civil twilight.

CLINICAL PEARL

Changes in outdoor illumination associated with sunrise and sunset produce sizable and selective changes in visual abilities, including visual acuity.

One obvious solution to offset this decline is to add artificial illumination by turning on one's automotive headlamps. Unfortunately, the intensity and the pattern of illumination provided by headlamps, particularly when used on the low beam setting, do not come close to compensating for the loss of illumination from the sun.[51] It would appear that even the so-called normally-sighted individual is, at nighttime and under adverse weather conditions, driving with degraded visual acuity.

It might, of course, be argued that the presence of a relatively normal visual field would compensate for the loss in visual acuity. However, there are at least three factors that weaken this argument. First, not all states test visual fields. Second, those individuals who wear a spectacle correction probably have, under the best of daytime conditions, a corrected field of view of closer to 90 or 100 degrees. Third, a driver with a normal visual system has a normal full visual field if and only if the pattern of environmental illumination is sufficient to support peripheral vision. Unfortunately, when driving at night and primarily by high beam headlamp illumination, the effective lateral field of view for the normally-sighted driver is only about 30 to 40 degrees.[51] Thus while a low vision patient having a similar visual field would probably be prevented from driving under the best of visibility conditions, there is no regulation or guideline that would prevent the normally-sighted from driving, even under the worst of visibility conditions. It is interesting to speculate that the vast majority of low vision driving is being done by the normally-sighted. From this perspective, the apparent success of a bioptic driving program[52] should not be very surprising.

CLINICAL PEARL

Automotive headlamps do not provide full compensation for the loss of vision associated with nightfall, even in the normally-sighted.

CLINICAL PEARL

It seems likely that most of the low vision driving is being done by normally-sighted individuals driving under visually impoverished conditions.

One important implication of this final section is the suggestion that state licensing agencies may be overestimating the visual requirements for safe, accident-free, driving. Normally-sighted individuals are able to drive safely across a wide range of conditions, including conditions under which their visual abilities can be presumed to be less than those of state vision standards. The results of Albert Burg and his successors are certainly consistent with this statement. Further, it was recently estimated that "a U.S. driver can expect to travel for 102 years before experiencing a disabling-injury accident, and one is not likely to fall victim to a fatal accident for 3738 years."[53]

In concluding this chapter, two points should be emphasized. One is that there will be an increasing number of elderly individuals who will face restriction or denial of licensure for failure to meet state vision standards. Accordingly, it would seem appropriate to base such action on empirically justifiable standards. Second, it should be clear that the mass-screening approach, by itself, will not provide the empirical evidence necessary to define those vision standards. Nor, for that matter, can such standards be defined by simply pointing out that the normally-sighted individuals do, at times, drive with impaired vision. Rather, new approaches are necessary, and new approaches are in fact being used to determine those aspects of the overall driving task that may depend selectively on different visual characteristics.[54-57]

CLINICAL PEARL

New experimental approaches are necessary to determine if existing vision standards for driver licensure can be relaxed without endangering public safety.

References

1. Transportation Research Board: *Transportation in an aging society: special report 218,* vol 1, Committee reports and recommendations, Washington, DC, 1988, National Research Council.
2. Transportation Research Board: *Transportation in an aging society: special report 218,* vol 2, Technical papers, Washington, DC, 1988, National Research Council.
3. Waller PF: The older driver, *Hum Factors* 33:499-505, 1991.
4. Kaszniak AW, Keyl PM, Albert MS: Dementia and the older driver, *Hum Factors* 33:527-538, 1991.
5. Parasuraman R, Nestor PG: Attention and driving skills in aging and Alzheimer's disease, *Hum Factors* 33:539-558, 1991.
6. Pitts DG: The effect of aging on selected visual functions. In Sekuler R, Klein D, Dismukes K (eds): *Aging and human visual function,* New York, 1982, Alan R Liss, 131-160.
7. Owsley C, Sloane ME: Vision and aging. In Boller F, Grafman J (eds): *Handbook of neuropsychology* vol 4, Amsterdam, 1990, Elsevier Science Publishers, 4:229-249.
8. National Eye Institute: *Vision research, a national plan: 1994-1998,* National Institutes of Health, Bethesda, Md.
9. Hills BJ: Vision, visibility, and perception in driving, *Perception* 9(2):183-216, 1980.
10. Shinar D, Schieber F: Visual requirements for safety and mobility of older drivers, *Hum Factors* 33:507-519, 1991.
11. Allen MJ: *Vision and highway safety,* Radnor, Pa, 1970, Chilton Book Co.
12. Freeman PB: Visual requirements for driving, *J Rehabil Optom* 2:6-7, Summer 1984.
13. Keltner JL, Johnson C: Visual function, driving safety, and the elderly, *Ophthalmology* 94:1180-1188, 1987.
14. National Highway Traffic Safety Administration and American Association of Motor Vehicle Administrators: State and provincial licensing systems, Department of Transportation, Washington, DC, 1985, US Government Printing Office.
15. Bailey IL, Sheedy JE: Vision screening for driver licensure, *Transportation in an Aging Society, Special Report 218* 2:294-324, 1988.
16. Appel S, Brilliant R, Reich L: Driving with visual impairment: facts and issues, *J Vis Rehabil* 4:19-31, 1990.
17. Higgins KE, Brilliant R, Appel S, Reich L, Briggs R, Leibowitz H: *Driving performance in the visually impaired individual,* Final report, National Institute on Disability and Rehabilitation Research, US Department of Education, 1990.
18. Fonda G: Bioptic telescopic spectacles for driving a motor vehicle, *Arch Ophthalmol* 92:348-349, 1974.
19. Keeney AH: Field loss vs central magnification: telescopes and the driving risk, *Arch Ophthalmol* 42:273, 1974.
20. Keeney AH, Weiss S, Silva D: Telescopic spectacles and motor vehicle driving licensure, *Trans Am Ophthalmol Soc* 70:261-264, 1972.
21. Keeney AH, Weiss S, Silva D: Functional problems of telescopic spectacles in the driving task, *Trans Am Ophthalmol Soc* 72:132-138, 1974.
22. Feinbloom W: Driving with bioptic telescopic spectacles, *Am J Optom Physiol Opt* 54:35-42, 1977.
23. Fonda G: Bioptic telescopic spectacle is a hazard for operating a motor vehicle? *Arch Ophthalmol* 101:1907-1908, 1983.
24. Bailey IL: Driving with bioptic telescopes: a position paper, *J Rehabil Optom* 2:9-11, Summer 1984.
25. Bailey IL: Bioptic telescopes, *Arch Ophthalmol* 103:13-14, 1985.
26. Kelleher DK: Driving with bioptics - a personal viewpoint, *J Rehabil Optom* 1:8-9, 1984.
27. Jose R, Carter K, Carter C: A training program for clients considering the use of bioptic telescopes for driving, *J Vis Impair Blindness* 77:425-428, 1983.

28. Jose R, Ousley BA: The visually handicapped, driving and bioptics - some new facts, *Rehabil Optom* 2:2-5, 1984.
29. Lippman O, Corn AL, Lewis MC: Bioptic telescopic spectacles and driving performance: a study in Texas, *J Vis Impair Blindness* 82:182-187, 1988.
30. Fonda G: Legal blindness can be compatible with safe driving, *Ophthalmology* 96:1457-1459, 1989.
31. Burg A: *The relationship between vision test scores and driving record: general findings*, Report 67-24, Department of Engineering, Los Angeles, 1967, University of California.
32. Burg A: *Vision test scores and driving record: additional findings*, Report 68-27, Department of Engineering, Los Angeles, 1968, University of California.
33. Burg A: Vision and driving. In Benson W, Whitcomb M (eds): *Current developments in optics and vision*, Washington, DC, 1968, National Academy of Sciences - National Research Council.
34. Runyon R, Haber A: *Fundamentals of behavioral statistics*, ed 6, New York, 1988, Random House.
35. Henderson RL, Burg A: *Vision and audition in driving*, US Department of Transportation, Report DOT-HS-801-265, Washington, DC, 1974, National Highway Administration.
36. Council FM, Allen JA: *Visual fields of North Carolina drivers and their relationship to accidents*, Chapel Hill, 1974, University of North Carolina, Highway Safety Research Center.
37. Shinar D: *Driver visual limitations diagnosis and treatment*, US Department of Transportation, Springfield, Va, 1977, National Technical Information Service.
38. Hills BJ, Burg A: *A re-analysis of California driver vision data: general findings*, Report 768, Crowthorne, England, 1977, Transport and Road Research Laboratory.
39. Keeney AH, Garvey JL, Brunker GF: *Current experience with the monocular drivers of Kentucky*, San Francisco, 1981, American Association of Automotive Medicine Proceedings.
40. Johnson CA, Keltner JL: Incidence of visual field loss on 20,000 eyes and its relationship to driving performance, *Arch Ophthalmol* 101(3):371-375, 1983.
41. Decina LE, Staplin L, Spiegel A: *Correcting unaware vision impaired drivers*, Contract No 730009, 1990, Pennsylvania Department of Transportation, Harrisburg, Pa.
42. Decina LE, Breton ME, Staplin L: *Visual disorders and commercial drivers*, Contract No DTFH61-90-C-00093, 1991, US Department of Transportation, Washington, DC.
43. Ball K, Owsley C: Identifying correlates of accident involvement for the older driver, *Hum Factors* 33:583-595, 1991.
44. Ball K, Owsley C, Sloane ME, Roenker DL, Bruni JR: Visual attention problems as a predictor of vehicle crashes in older drivers, *Invest Ophthalmol Vis Sci* 34:3110-3123, 1993.
45. Bailey IL, Sheedy JE: Vision and the aging driver. In Cole RG, Rosenthal BP (eds): *Problems in Optometry* 4(1):59-71, 1992.
46. Graham C: *Vision and visual perception*, New York, 1965, John Wiley & Sons, Inc.
47. Johnson CA: Peripheral visual functions at various adaptation levels. In *Night vision: current research and future directions*, Washington, DC, 1987, National Academy Press, 256-274.
48. Owsley C: Aging and night vision. In *Night vision: current research and future directions*, Washington, DC, 1987, National Academy Press, 275-287.
49. Leibowitz HW, Owens DA: We drive by night: and when we do, we often misjudge our visual capabilities, courting disaster, *Psychology Today* 20:55-58, 1986.
50. Leibowitz HW, Owens DA: Can normal outdoor activities be carried out during civil twilight? *Applied Optics* 30(24):3501-3503, 1991.
51. Owens DA, Francis E, Leibowitz HW: Visibility distance with headlights: a functional approach, Technical Paper No 890684, 1989, Society of Automotive Engineering, Warrendale, Pa.

52. Janke M, Kazarian G: *The accident record of drivers with bioptic telescopic lenses*, Report 86, Sacramento, 1983, State of California, Department of Motor Vehicles.
53. Owens DA, Helmers G, Sivak M: Intelligent vehicle highway systems: a call for user-centered design, *Ergonomics* 36:363-369, 1993.
54. Wood JM, Troutbeck R: Effect of restriction of the binocular visual field on driving performance, *Ophthalmic Physiol Opt* 12:291-298, 1992.
55. Wood JM, Troutbeck R: The effect of visual impairment on driving, *Hum Factors* 36:476-487, 1994.
56. Wood JM, Troutbeck R: The effect of artificial visual impairment on functional visual fields and driving performance, *Clin Vis Sci*, 8:563-575, 1993.
57. Szlyk JP, Alexander KR, Severing K, Fishman G: Assessment of driving performance in patients with retinitis pigmentosa, *Arch Opthalmol* 110:1709-1713, 1992.

11

Typography, Print Legibility, and Low Vision

Aries Arditi

Key Terms

legibility	letter stroke width	crowding
reading acuity	letter aspect ratio	Americans with
typography	letter spacing	Disabilities Act

The loss of ability to read is well known to be one of the most disabling functional problems experienced by those with low vision,[1] and providing renewed access to text after vision loss is a focal task of vision rehabilitation.

Most methods for remediating reduced access to text in low vision employ magnification, because increasing optical size of letter and word patterns and distributing their information over a larger retinal area is highly effective in increasing the ability to identify visual patterns. Magnification may be done optically at the eye, or environmentally at the text stimulus (as with large print and signage).

It is so effective and consistent a visual aid that pattern processing capability itself is often characterized by the amount of image magnification an individual requires for effective visual processing. Thus using standard letter optotypes as patterns, *letter acuity* measurements identify the minimum retinal size an individual requires for reliable letter identification. Similarly, *reading acuity* measurements use standard fonts to identify the minimum retinal size an individual requires for reading. In this way, relative magnification of just discriminable standard stimuli is used to characterize the visual resolving capabilities of patients.

Magnification can also be used in a similar way to characterize the relative discriminability, legibility, or readability of text fonts and optotypes. In other words, rather than using standard optotypes and fonts to assess observers, visual acuity itself can be used to access relative legibility, by comparing acuities obtained under different typographic conditions within research subjects. Compared to other measures of legibility such as reading speed,[2,3] reading acuity is an appropriate measure of legibility in the context of low vision, since so many low vision patients must read letter by letter, at their acuity limit.

CLINICAL PEARL

Visual acuity itself can be used to access relative legibility, by comparing acuities obtained under different typographic conditions within research subjects.

CLINICAL PEARL

Reading acuity is an appropriate measure of legibility in the context of low vision, since so many low vision patients must read letter by letter, at their acuity limit.

Using such acuity methods, we have recently begun to identify general characteristics of letter forms and typography that make text more or less readable, and optotypes more or less legible. Previous attempts to study text legibility parametrically have lacked generality, using only one or two numeral forms at a time, and testing perceptibility[4-6] or exposure duration[7] rather than letter discrimination.

We use a font design program, written in the METAFONT[8] computer language, whose parameters may be independently adjusted to produce a family of fonts that vary in selected ways thought to have strong effects on legibility: stroke width, letter spacing, and width-to-height (aspect) ratio. This program also generates the Sloan letters used in the Lighthouse/ETDRS acuity chart and the British letters used in the Bailey-Lovie chart with suitable adjustment of parameters. The Sloan letters are among those in the upper row of Figure 11-1.

Generally, our methods are to present random five-letter text strings using the fonts of interest on an optically minified CRT, which brings the text on the display close to the acuity limit. If the observer

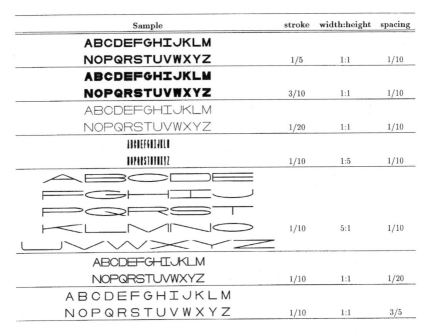

Sample	stroke	width:height	spacing
ABCDEFGHIJKLM NOPQRSTUVWXYZ	1/5	1:1	1/10
ABCDEFGHIJKLM NOPQRSTUVWXYZ	3/10	1:1	1/10
ABCDEFGHIJKLM NOPQRSTUVWXYZ	1/20	1:1	1/10
ABCDEFGHIJKLM NOPQRSTUVWXYZ	1/10	1:5	1/10
ABCDEFGHIJ KLMNO PQRST UVWXYZ	1/10	5:1	1/10
ABCDEFGHIJKLM NOPQRSTUVWXYZ	1/10	1:1	1/20
A B C D E F G H I J K L M N O P Q R S T U V W X Y Z	1/10	1:1	3/5

FIGURE 11-1 Font samples illustrating several typographic parameters. The first three samples differ only in stroke width; the fourth and fifth samples differ only in width-to-height ratio; the sixth and last samples differ only in interletter spacing. Stroke width and spacing are expressed in units of letter height.

identifies all five letters correctly, the text is reduced in size by 0.05 log unit; if at least one letter is incorrectly identified, the letter size is increased by 0.05 log unit. After 24 reversals of this psychophysical staircase, the average text size of letters presented is computed, and represents the 90% correct identification threshold. For comparison to visual acuity data, this size can be presented as the minimum angle of resolution (MAR), conventionally defined as $\frac{1}{5}$ the letter height.

Letter Stroke Width

Figure 11-2 shows how legibility (as measured by letter acuity) varies as a function of stroke width for each of five subjects, and for each of three letter spacings (parameter).[9] The fonts used were among the family shown in Figure 11-1 with 1:1 width-to-height ratio. For the widest spaced letters (triangles), legibility is an inverted U-shaped function of stroke width, with very thin and very thick letters being more difficult to identify. It is reasonable to suppose that the thickest stroked letters become less legible because gaps and other features that distinguish the letters are more difficult to resolve (Figure 11-1, row 2). Effects of letter spacing on thinner stroked letters are discussed later.

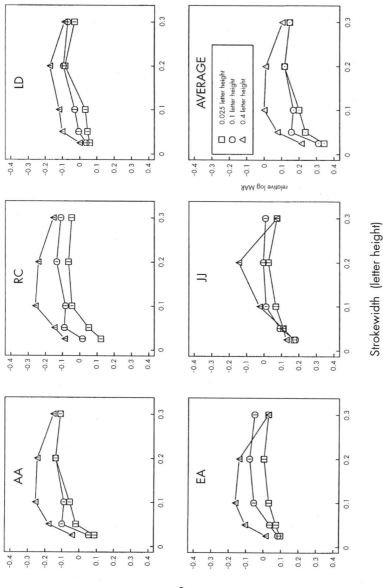

FIGURE 11-2 Legibility expressed as log MAR, as a function of letter stroke width for five subjects and three spacings (shown in the inset in the lower right panel). Average data are shown as departures from maximum legibility. Standard error bars are shown only for individual subject's data. (From Arditi A et al: Letter strokewidth, spacing, and legibility. In *Vision science and its applications*, vol 1, OSA Technical Digest Series, Washington, DC, 1995, Optical Society of America, 324-327.

One of the most interesting aspects of these data is that there is a range encompassing at least an octave (0.1 to 0.2 letter height) of stroke widths in which there is little (less than 0.1 log MAR, equivalent to one chart line) variation in legibility. While this seems to be true for these normal observers, low vision patients, especially those with reduced contrast sensitivity due to ocular media opacities and reduced retinal illuminances, may have particular difficulty with thinly stroked letter forms,[10] because they contain less contrast energy than do thickly stroked letters.

CLINICAL PEARL

There is a range encompassing at least an octave (0.1 to 0.2 letter height) of stroke widths in which there is little (less than 0.1 log MAR, equivalent to one chart line) variation in legibility.

CLINICAL PEARL

Low vision patients, especially those with reduced contrast sensitivity due to ocular media opacities and reduced retinal illuminances, may have particular difficulty with thinly stroked letter forms

---

Letter Form Aspect Ratio

The width-to-height ratio of letter forms also has a strong impact on legibility as defined by minimum discriminable size (Figure 11-3).[11] In this case, where the aspect ratio varies, minimum size is not easily characterized. In the figure, the data are plotted in three ways: column A as a function of minimum vertical size, column B minimum horizontal size, and column C minimum vertical or horizontal size, whichever is greater. Expressed as in *A*, legibility increases with width-to-height ratio throughout the range of aspect ratios from 0.2 to 5, whereas it decreases throughout the same range, when expressed as in *B*. Both *A* and *B* indicate that adding horizontal *or* vertical extent to letter forms has an effect on legibility throughout this range of aspect ratios, although the direction of the effect depends on what measure of letter size is used. Rows 4 and 5 of Figure 11-1 illustrate the extremes of the aspect ratios tested in Figure 11-3. In this experiment, each aspect ratio tested other than unity had a counterpart with reciprocally-valued aspect ratio that was also tested (e.g., 0.2 and 5).

Figure 11-3 exhibits an interesting asymmetry, most apparent in the right-hand column of the graphs. Fonts with width-to-height ratios less than unity are consistently more legible than their counterparts

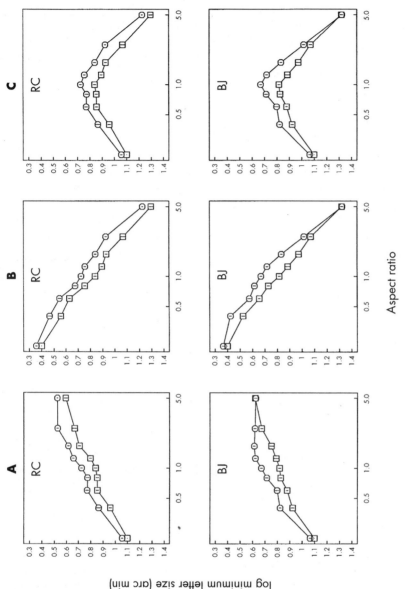

FIGURE 11-3 Legibility measured as log minimum letter size, as a function of letter width-to-height ratio, for two subjects, at two interletter spacings (squares: 0.05 letter height, circles: 2 letter height). **Column A,** plots log minimum vertical size of letters. **Column B,** plots log minimum horizontal size of letters. **Column C,** plots log minimum size of the larger (vertical or horizontal) dimension.

with reciprocal aspect ratio. This may be due to the greater amount of vertical than horizontal information distinguishing uppercase letters in the spatial-frequency bands used in the acuity discrimination.

CLINICAL PEARL

Fonts with width-to-height ratios less than unity are consistently more legible than their counterparts with reciprocal aspect ratio.

Letter Spacing

A third typographic variable of interest is that of interletter spacing. Acuity for letters or optotypes presented in close proximity to other letters [2,12,13,14,15] or other contours [13,16] is widely known to be significantly worse than it is for isolated letter or optotype forms. Such deficits, known as "crowding" phenomena, have been found to be worse in amblyopia and in disorders of the central visual field,[13,15,16,17,18] and thus may have special relevance to low vision.

Close spacing has also been shown to reduce reading speed at letter sizes close to the acuity limit,[2] but not with larger letters.[2,3] With larger letters, close spacing actually improves reading speeds,[19] probably because eye movement requirements for reading such text are more modest.[2]

Given the substantial literature on crowding phenomena, it is not surprising that close spacing also results in reduced acuity for text strings. This is demonstrated in Figure 11-2, which also plots effects of stroke width on acuity. What is of particular interest about these data is that for the two closer and less legible spacings shown in the figure (0.1 and 0.025 letter height), legibility does not suffer so much when letters are very thickly stroked, as it does for the wider spacing (0.4 letter height). With close spacing, small gaps probably do not serve as such effective marks to distinguish letters since they exist between and within letters. Additionally, with close spacing the letters are more difficult to localize than they are when separated by more space.

Figure 11-4 shows the same data as Figure 11-2, replotted to emphasize effects of spacing on legibility. In general the effects of spacing (crowding) are similar for all stroke widths except the thickest, where wide spacing fails to offer an advantage.

CLINICAL PEARL

Effects of spacing (crowding) are similar for all stroke widths except the thickest, where wide spacing fails to offer an advantage.

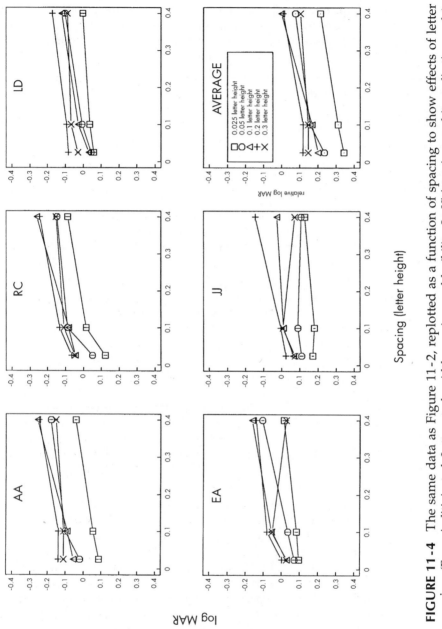

FIGURE 11-4 The same data as Figure 11-2, replotted as a function of spacing to show effects of letter spacing. (From Arditi A et al: Letter strokewidth, spacing, and legibility. In *Vision science and its applications*, vol 1, OSA Technical Digest Series, Washington, DC, 1995, Optical Society of America, 324-327.

At ARVO in 1993[20] and at the International Low Vision Conference in 1993,[10] we proposed that crowding phenomena were simply an instance of lateral masking of the target letter by neighboring contours. We hypothesized that since spatial masking occurs predominantly within spatial-frequency bands, crowding phenomena should depend on the spectral composition of the target and neighboring forms. Since the Fourier spectra of thickly stroked letters have more energy at lower object spatial frequencies than do thinly stroked letters, they can exert a masking influence over a larger neighboring region. Our finding that crowding effects are no greater for thickly stroked than for thinly stroked letters suggests that contrary to our earlier beliefs, crowding is not an instance of spatial-frequency dependent lateral masking. It is also possible that crowding is an instance of lateral masking, but that information critical to letter identification at the acuity limit exists within a fixed object spatial-frequency band.

As to potential interactions between aspect ratio and letter spacing, the data of Figure 11-3 do not show any evidence for them. That is, spacing and aspect ratio seem to have independent effects on legibility.

CLINICAL PEARL

Spacing and aspect ratio seem to have independent effects on legibility.

Other Typographic Variables

There are many other typographic variables that can affect legibility of text. Arditi, Knoblauch, and Grunwald[2] found proportionally spaced fonts to be more legible than fixed space fonts at most character sizes, but found fixed space fonts to be more legible at retinal sizes close to the acuity limit. Morris et al.[21] also found proportionally spaced fonts to be superior to fixed space at sufficient sizes, and Mansfield et al[22] replicated Arditi et al's results at the acuity limit.

Italics, slanted fonts, and decorative/ornate styles are all thought to be less legible,[23,24] but this probably has less to do with their physical characteristics than with readers' relative lack of familiarity with the letter forms.

Many studies of reading performance have focused on the role of contrast.[3,25,26] All are consistent with the views that increasing contrast never decreases legibility, and that it generally increases legibility for patients with effective contrast reductions due to pathology, and for normally-sighted individuals viewing low contrast text. In addition, there is some evidence that for patients who report significant problems with glare, white text on a black background is more legible than the reverse, presumably because the amount of light entering the eye in the region of the text is lower in the former case than in the latter. Thus for designers of text displays, maximum legibility for the largest proportion of the normally-sighted and visually impaired population seems to be achieved with the highest feasible contrasts, using white letters on a dark background.

What color combinations result in the highest text readability? The few studies that have addressed this issue[27,28] have in general found that the most important chromatic determinant of readability is the luminosity contrast component of the color combination comprising the letters and background of the text display. In other words, for the standard observer (with a standard spectral luminosity function), hue and saturation per se are irrelevant—the luminance contrast between the colors chosen for letters and background alone determines the readability. Of course, relative to the standard observer most low vision patients have some color defect, either congenital or acquired through aging or disorders producing spectrally nonuniform ocular media opacities or selective cone losses. These color defects often result in luminosity functions that differ markedly from the standard observer. As a result, some color combinations produce higher effective contrasts and hence higher readability than others for these observers.

Further discussion of this issue and a set of three simple rules for optimizing color contrast are contained in a chapter by Arditi and Knoblauch entitled *Effective color contrast and low vision* that appears in the companion to this volume.[29] Also, nontechnical brochures describing 10 guidelines for increasing print legibility and how to compose effective color contrasts for partially-sighted individuals are available free from The Lighthouse Inc.[23,30]

The Role of Typography in Vision Rehabilitation

As noted earlier, amelioration of vision loss may be provided proximally to the eye, as with an optical or optoelectronic magnifier, or environmentally, by large print or large signage. Proximal vision aids that increase the retinal size of the visual stimulus are generally more portable and more easily adjustable to the patient's individual needs as far as focus, field of view, lighting level, etc.

But magnification alone is often insufficient to provide successful access to text in some reading situations, particularly outside the home (e.g., reading signs) where adjustments of light, magnification, and viewing distance cannot be easily controlled by the patient. Although telescopic aids can be used in such situations, they are difficult to use effectively and often require a great deal of skill and training.[31] Furthermore, magnification range is generally more limited since the devices must be handheld or headmounted and are therefore more susceptible to hand and head tremor. Increasing text size environmentally may also be infeasible due to limited sign space or economic constraints (e.g., size and/or number of pages in a large print book).

The Americans with Disabilities Act (ADA) of 1990 has recognized the importance of visual signage enhancement in its Title III Guidelines for Buildings and Facilities (ADAAG) published July 21, 1991.[32] The ADAAG, which addresses public accommodations and commercial facilities,* has, for various types of signs, requirements that are intended to provide increased legibility by means of specifying ranges of type style, letter size, proportion and stroke width, sign finish, and a recommended contrast minimum. Unfortunately, these guidelines were written without sufficient research to specify such ranges with confidence.

One reason why such research has been lacking is that until recently, ability to vary typographic parameters was costly, and there was little need to specify in general terms the effects of typographic variation on legibility. With the advent of computerized typography,[33] infinite variations of typefaces are very easy to implement. This makes it easy to abuse typography, and at the same time allows the study of how general typographic parameters affect text legibility, and the potential for customizing typography for maximum legibility for persons with low vision.

References

1. Faye EE: *Clinical low vision*, ed 2, Boston, 1984, Little, Brown & Co.
2. Arditi A, Knoblauch K, Grunwald I: Reading with fixed and variable character pitch, *J Opt Soc Am* 7A:2011-2015, 1990.
3. Legge GE, Rubin GS, Pelli DG, Schleske MM: Psychophysics of reading. II. Low vision, *Vision Res* 25(2):253–266, 1985.
4. Berger C: Stroke-width, form and horizontal spacing of numerals as determinants of the threshold of recognition, I, *J Appl Psychol* 28:208-231, 1944.
5. Berger C: Stroke-width, form and horizontal spacing of numerals as determinants of the threshold of recognition, II, *J Appl Psychol* 28:336-346, 1944.
6. Berger C: Experiments on the legibility of symbols of different width and height, *Acta Ophthalmol* 26:423-434, 1948.
7. Soar RS: Height-width proportion and stroke width in numerical visibility, *J Appl Psychol* 39:43-46, 1955.
8. Knuth DE: *The METAFONTbook,* American Mathematical Society, Reading, Mass, 1986, Addison-Wesley.
9. Arditi A, Cagenello R, Jacobs B: Letter Strokewidth, spacing, and legibility. In *Vision science and its applications*, vol 1, OSA Technical Digest Series, Washington, DC, 1995, Optical Society of America, 324-327.

---

* These terms have technical meanings that are too lengthy to describe here, but which cover a wide range of privately operated and privately owned business facilities, and facilities that provide goods and services to the public.

10. Arditi A: On the relationship of letter acuity to reading acuity. In Kooijman AC, Looijestijn PL, Welling JA, van der Wildt GJ (eds): *Low vision: research and new developments in rehabilitation*, Amsterdam, 1994, IOS Press, 38-45.

11. Arditi A, Cagenello R, Jacobs B: Effects of aspect ratio and spacing on legibility of small letters, *Invest Ophthalmol Vis Sci* 36(4):671, 1995.

12. Anstis SM: A chart demonstrating variations in acuity with retinal position, *Vision Res* 14:589-592, 1974.

13. Flom MC, Weymouth FW, Kahneman, D: Visual resolution and contour interaction, *J Opt Soc Am* 53:1026-1032, 1963.

14. Skottun BC, Freeman RD: Perceived size of letters depends on interletter spacing: a new visual illusion, *Vision Res* 23:111-12, 1983.

15. Stuart JA, Burian HM: A study of separation difficulty: its relationship to visual acuity in normal and amblyopic eyes, *Am J Ophthalmol* 53:471-477, 1962.

16. Loomis JM: Lateral masking in foveal and eccentric vision, *Vision Res* 18:335-338, 1978.

17. Bouma H: Interaction effects in parafoveal letter recognition, *Nature* 226:177-178, 1970.

18. Whittaker S, Rohrskaste F, Higgins K: Optimum letter spacing for word recognition in central and eccentric fields. In *Digest of topical meeting on noninvasive assessment of the visual system*, Washington, DC, 1989, Optical Society of America, 56-59.

19. Moriarty SE, Scheiner EC: A study of close-set text type, *J Appl Psychol* 69:700-702, 1984.

20. Arditi A, Cagenello R: Why reading acuity is worse than and is poorly predicted by letter acuity, *Invest Ophthalmol Vis Sci* 34:1417, 1993.

21. Morris RA, Berry K, Hargreaves K, Liarakopis, D: How typeface variation and typographic scaling affect readability at small sizes. In Pennington K, Pietrowski K (eds): *IS&T's seventh international congress on advances in non-impact printing technologies*, Portland, Ore, 1991, Society for Imaging Science and Technology.

22. Mansfield JS, Legge GE, Cunningham K, Luebker A: The effect of font on reading-speed and reading-acuity in normal and low vision, *Invest Ophthalmol Vis Sci* 35:1554, 1994.

23. Arditi A: *Print legibility and partial sight*, New York, 1994, The Lighthouse Research Institute.

24. Tinker MA: *Legibility of print*, Ames, Iowa, 1963, Iowa State University Press.

25. Legge GE, Pelli DG, Rubin GS, Schleske MM: Psychophysics of reading. I. Normal vision, *Vision Res* 25:239-252, 1985.

26. Legge GE, Rubin GS, Schleske MM: Psychophysics of reading. V. The role of contrast in normal vision, *Vision Res* 27:1165-1177, 1985.

27. Knoblauch K, Arditi A, Szlyk, J: Effects of chromatic and luminance contrast on reading, *J Opt Soc Am* 8A:428-439, 1991.

28. Legge GE, Parish DH, Luebker A, Wurm LH: Psychophysics of reading. XI. Comparing luminance and color contrast, *J Opt Soc Am* 7A:2002-2010, 1990.

29. Arditi A, Knoblauch K: Effective color contrast and low vision. In Rosenthal B, Cole R (eds): *Functional assessment of low vision*, St Louis, 1995, Mosby.

30. Arditi A: *Color contrast and partial sight: how to design with colors that contrast effectively for people with low vision and color deficiencies*, New York, 1995, The Lighthouse Research Institute.

31. Jose RT: *Understanding low vision*, New York, 1983, American Foundation for the Blind.

32. Architectural and Transportation Barriers Compliance Board: Americans with disabilities act (ADA) accessibility guidelines for buildings and facilities, final guidelines, 36 CFR Part 1191, *Fed Reg* 56(44):35407-35542, 1991.

33. Rubenstein R: *Digital typography: an introduction to type and composition for computer system design*, Reading, Mass, 1988, Addison-Wesley Publishing Co.

12

Considerations in Establishing Low Vision Care

Karen R. Seidman
Clare M. Hood

Key Terms

low vision care	vision rehabilitation	low vision practice
comprehensive low	vision impairment	management
vision care		

Low vision care is practiced throughout the United States in eye care settings including solo practices, single-specialty and multi-specialty groups, hospital clinics, and vision rehabilitation agencies. In the United States alone there are nearly 200 clinics identified where low vision care is offered[1] and many more private practice settings now include this growing specialty of ophthalmology and optometry. Increasing numbers of clinicians are asking, should I provide low vision care? and, how does one get started in this specialty?

The answer to the first question is clear. Current statistics show that over 10 million people—about 1 out of every 20 in the United States—have a significant impairment of vision which cannot be further improved by corrective lenses, surgery, or medication, and are potential candidates for low vision rehabilitation. Almost 13% of all noninstitutionalized people 65 years of age or over report a vision impairment, and this percentage grows as we consider those between the ages of 75 and 84 (16%) and those 85 years of age or over (27%).[2] We are looking toward an even more striking demand for low vision services as the baby boom generation ages and experiences the range of age related eye diseases. Demographers tell us that there will be unprecedented growth in the number of older people in our population, and project that by the year 2020 there will be 4.6 million older adults with vision impairments.[3] This, coupled with medical advances in neonatal care, point to a dramatic increase in the number of people across the life span who may seek low vision care.

CLINICAL PEARL

We are looking toward an even more striking demand for low vision services as the baby boom generation ages and experiences the range of age related eye diseases.

In addition to the growing demand, developments within the field of low vision care should be encouraging to those who want to add this specialty. The evolution of this clinical practice has made it possible to provide high-level, quality care in many settings for the person with impaired vision. A structured examination procedure has replaced "trial and error" in the assessment of residual vision. A battery of function tests yields quantitative and qualitative information that can be useful as a predictor of optical devices and patients' responses. Optical equipment is varied and readily available. Specialized vision rehabilitation is available in the community. Some funding sources exist, and new professionals joining the low vision team are enhancing service delivery. All of these advances are fueled by the availability of continuing professional education in low vision care.

Comprehensive Low Vision Care

How to get started in low vision care is not quite as obvious as the need. This stems in part from the challenges imposed by the wide variation in potential service delivery models. Designing a low vision specialty practice starts with the recognition that each setting represents different needs and will require different strategies. However, making a commitment to achieving comprehensive low vision care, whether provided entirely from within one's own practice, or by utilizing other available resources and service providers, is a crucial first step.

> **CLINICAL PEARL**
>
> *Making a commitment to achieving comprehensive low vision care, whether provided entirely from within one's own practice, or by utilizing other available resources and service providers, is a crucial first step.*

The following components are fundamental to comprehensive low vision care. They should be considered in the planning process and a determination made as to where and by whom they will be provided.

1. Diagnostic eye care
2. Medical treatment/surgery for eye disease
3. Analysis of visual function
4. Discussion of the visual tasks in the patient's daily life
5. Low vision examination
6. Assessment of the psychosocial factors affected by vision loss
7. Provision of a range of optical equipment for testing/loan/ dispensing
8. Instruction in the use of optical devices and recommendation of adaptive/assistive devices
9. Prescription of these devices.
10. Dispensing of devices
11. Patient education for awareness of existing community resources
12. Vision rehabilitation services, and other specialized rehabilitation
13. Access to available funding sources for services/devices
14. Continuing eye care
15. Training and continuing education for clinicians and staff

Many combinations may be effective in securing comprehensive low vision care for patients. In your own clinical setting, one or more of the following important components may be provided: primary eye care, low vision evaluation/prescription/dispensing, patient education, referral for and/or additional resources/services, and specialized vision rehabilitation. You may decide to offer low vision optical care in-house and to request consultation for other rehabilitation or educational services from a private or state vision rehabilitation agency, hospital, or school. You may choose to refer patients to low vision specialists in your community and offer resource information only. These decisions will dictate many things about the way you set up your practice, including space to be designated, staff to be involved, scheduling, equipment needs, and plans for follow-up care.

Once you have decided to offer low vision care, preparation involves: (1) identifying other low vision and rehabilitation services in your community, (2) identifying the scope of the low vision services you intend to offer, (3) establishing the surroundings and atmosphere which support the examination/instruction/dispensing procedures by reviewing the office environment and the office routine, (4) identifying staff roles and the need for additional clinician and staff education, (5) rewriting job descriptions and adjusting salaries, (6) integrating the specialty into your billing system, and (7) developing/ acquiring appropriate resource information and consultation sources. Attention to these steps in your advance preparation will allow you to make a realistic plan for introducing low vision care into your practice setting, and to obtain appropriate optical, testing, and other equipment in a cost effective and timely way.

CLINICAL PEARL

Reviewing the office environment (color, contrast, accessibility), the office routine (scheduling, forms, resource information), and providing staff education about special needs of people with impaired vision will help in the planning and delivery of low vision care.

Reviewing the Office Environment

Anticipating the needs of persons with low vision is an important stage in the process of getting ready to offer low vision care. Many modifications you choose to incorporate may be appreciated by your other patients, as well.

Take a walk with your office manager and look at the places low vision patients will use. Consider their accessibility. Some elements of the Americans with Disabilities Act Accessibility Guidelines are relevant to people with impaired vision.[4] These guidelines provide minimum standards for new construction, but there are additional enhancements that you can make right now to improve your practice's accessibility for people who have low vision.

Are elevator buttons/floors well marked? Can an elderly person manage to get into and out of waiting room and examination chairs? Can wheelchairs and walkers be accommodated? Is there room for family members or friends who have accompanied patients to join them in examination or instruction areas? Look at the color schemes. Is there adequate contrast in the colors you have chosen so that patients can distinguish the furniture from the floor, doors from walls, etc.?[5] Do white fixtures in rest rooms disappear against white tiles? Is there adequate, adjustable lighting in the waiting room so that patients can read or fill out the forms you will require? Is there a selection of large print popular reading material in the waiting room?

Consider the space to be used for the actual low vision examination/ instruction/dispensing. Will a unique space be dedicated for this, or (more likely) will you schedule room(s) for low vision as needed? There are advantages to separating the room used for examination from the instruction space, but alternate approaches are feasible when space is limited. Remember that you will need storage space for the low vision optical and nonoptical devices and a file of resource information including patient education pamphlets, catalogues and directories. If lenses to loan and to dispense will be components of your service, additional equipment, storage space, and record keeping will be needed.

Reviewing the Office Routine

In addition to looking at the office environment, consider the office routine on different days and at different times of day. It can be very helpful to make rounds of the office to observe the patient flow in preparation for making scheduling decisions as you prepare to add a low vision specialty. Rather than trying to squeeze low vision care appointments into any regular office day, it is most helpful (for doctor, staff, and patients) to reserve a day or part of a day specifically for low vision examinations and instruction. Consider the members of the staff who are likely to be involved with the low vision patient during a routine initial or follow-up visit and block out time for each of them to work. Reviewing the patient flow and scheduling accurately will help to avert uncomfortable situations for the patient and tension for the staff.

CLINICAL PEARL

Rather than trying to squeeze low vision care appointments into any regular office day, it is most helpful (for doctor, staff, and patients) to reserve a day or part of a day specifically for low vision examinations and instruction.

Think about the referral criteria for a patient to enter your low vision practice. If you plan to see patients referred by your colleagues in other practices, do they know what your referral criteria are? What type of referral document will they use? Even in group practices, where one doctor in the group will provide low vision care for the patients of the group, a referral document should be considered and referral criteria made clear. Early referrals—so effective in successful low vision care—are encouraged by specifying to ophthalmological and optometric colleagues the functional criteria for referral along with acuity criteria. Add to the office's resource file the directories of services that will be necessary for consultations and referrals.

Review your office's medical emergency procedures and equipment. Also review procedures for infection control, especially as they relate to lenses for testing and loan.

Consider the forms that may need to be developed or modified for each of the professionals who will work with the low vision patient. A variety of examination forms is currently available for the clinician to review and adapt.[6,7] Prepare to make the print legible on forms to be read by patients, such as appointment cards, releases, directions to the office, and insurance notices. Photo enlarging on a copier is often all that is necessary. When original documents are prepared, research indicates that using upper and lower case type in 16 to 18 point size is easiest for the majority of people with low vision to read. Spacing between lines should be at least 25% to 30% of the point size.[8]

Education for Staff

The decision to add the specialty of low vision care to the practice often will result in the need for additional staff education. Usually this will be continuing professional education in the techniques of examination, instruction, and dispensing for those who will provide direct care for the patient. However, don't forget the administrative staff. They will be better prepared to understand the implications of the new specialty for their own job duties if in-service education is provided.

In many practice settings, discussions with all members of the office staff take place well in advance of the addition of a new service. This can help to crystallize the practice's commitment to the new group of patients to be served. In the case of low vision care, these discussions allow staff to express their feelings about working with patients who have irreversible vision loss, and to think about and suggest modifications they may need to make in their own job activities. In most cases the modifications are simple, but can enhance the way the patient feels about the practice. For example, staff can have dark felt-tipped pens, signature guides, and adjustable lighting available for patients to sign forms more easily. They can provide directions in large print and be explicit in giving spoken directions for getting from one part of the office to another. In addition, they can learn proper "sighted guide" techniques to offer appropriate assistance when needed. These techniques improve the interaction between patients and staff, and underscore the fact that the practice is concerned about its patients with low vision.

Continuing professional education in low vision care is available from a number of different sources. Information can be obtained from the American Academy of Optometry, the American Optometric Association, the American Academy of Ophthalmology, local and state optometric associations, and the professional and continuing education programs of colleges of optometry. The Joint Commission on Allied Health Personnel in Ophthalmology provides information on accredited courses in low vision assisting, and the American Society of Ophthalmic Registered Nurses includes low vision in its regional and national training agendas. Other settings in which low vision clinical care is practiced (e.g., community hospitals) may also offer lectures. The Lighthouse Inc., in New York provides basic and advanced low vision courses, advanced case conferences, and practice management consultations.[9]

Integrating Low Vision Care into Your Billing System

While the decision to offer low vision care may arise from your commitment to comprehensive eye care or your desire to keep pace with the demand of your patients, the economic implications of your decision are important. Unfortunately, vision rehabilitation does not currently enjoy equal stature with physical rehabilitation, either in the reimbursement structure or the ease of patients' timely referral from the treatment phase to the restoration of function through use of compensatory devices, techniques, and strategies. Maximizing the return for services and/or devices is not as simple as getting used to the requirements of one carrier or learning a few procedure codes. It requires an understanding of multiple carriers and sponsors, and a knowledge of the unique provisions of coverage for persons with impaired vision. It also requires an understanding of local or regional policy and special programs for which patients may be eligible based on their particular situations. Most of all, it requires mastery of time efficient and cost effective low vision examination and instruction procedures.

CLINICAL PEARL

Unfortunately, vision rehabilitation does not currently enjoy equal stature with physical rehabilitation, either in the reimbursement structure or the ease of patients' timely referral from the treatment phase to the restoration of function through use of compensatory devices, techniques, and strategies.

Despite this complex scenario, there are several payment sources to consider. These include Medicare, Medicaid, state services for the blind and visually handicapped, state offices of vocational rehabilitation, private insurance carriers, plans for the military and their dependents, managed care and capitation plans, local service organizations, and of course, patient payments. Understandably, clinicians are most interested in Medicare coverage, since the 65 and over age group represents the bulk of the low vision population in any general practice.

Although the Health Care Financing Administration has acknowledged that significant vision loss may be recognized as a physical impairment, [10] there is no unique coding for a low vision examination or for the specialized vision rehabilitation services which may enhance vision device use and patients' functioning. Regional interpretation of low vision care varies widely among Medicare carriers. However, a range of evaluation and management codes may be considered for certain eye care services offered for the particular billable diagnoses. Since the therapeutic process leading to the prescription of low vision optical treatment varies significantly in different settings, *exploration with your carrier is essential.* The carrier's interpretation of existing evaluation and management codes within the context of the way you deliver, or plan to deliver, this type of eye care is the best way to clarify potential reimbursement pathways under Medicare. It is important to remember that Medicare does not routinely provide any coverage for low vision devices, although there has been one instance (1994) in which Medicare funds were authorized on appeal for a video magnifier (CCTV).

State rehabilitation services are particularly important in the low vision reimbursement picture. Low vision clinicians may find that examinations, follow-up care, and/or low vision devices for eligible patients may be funded in full or in part through state services for the blind and visually impaired. The entity that administers these programs in each state will vary, as will the extent of the services covered, and the participation and reporting requirements. Awareness of these programs is important to the practice that offers low vision care. Along with local private agencies, state rehabilitation programs are a resource to which the office can refer eligible patients for a range of rehabilitation and counseling services. They may also represent a source of referrals for low vision care and a potential source of coverage for services rendered.

It is clear that Medicare, state services, and other plans may be important to the reimbursement structure for your practice. To guide you in making the best use of each plan, begin by asking yourself several questions about **your** low vision services. Then, ask questions to gather the information you will need about the specifics of each plan, in order to evaluate its potential and its impact on your practice. Questions about the practice include the following:

- Will referrals for consultation be accepted from clinicians outside the practice, or will only patients of the practice be seen?
- If any additional providers will be added to offer this care, will they be part of the basic provider group or separately established?

- Will additional medical/optometric personnel work with the patient? Are they licensed/certified in their respective specialties?
- What procedures will comprise the office visit?
- Will dispensing of optical devices be handled on the premises or elsewhere?

Questions for carriers include the following:

- What are the requirements in order to be a provider of services within the particular reimbursement plan? Is it necessary for the provider to make a special application, to pass a qualifying examination, to show proof of continuing education to sign a contract or letter of agreement, etc.? Does participation in the plan influence the fee for services or devices?
- What codes apply to your particular setting, specialty, patient population, and services?
- Are any fees billable to the patient, and is any documentation necessary in order to do this?
- Are there any restrictions or requirements inherent in particular procedure codes?
- Is a fee schedule for services and devices available from the carrier?
- Is there a listing of maximum reimbursable amounts for services/devices or a charge report detailing approved reimbursement levels for relevant services or visits?
- How does the carrier calculate the amount to be paid to the provider?
- What are the timing requirements or guidelines for providers to submit claims and to receive payments?
- Does the carrier make written material available concerning the billing process?
- Are there seminars run by the carrier that you can attend to clarify billing questions?

You may find that you already have some of the references useful for coding information, including the CPT[11] (*Physicians' Current Procedural Terminology*), and the ICD-9-CM[12] (*International Classification of Diseases, 9th Revision*). A comprehensive listing of state rehabilitation services can be found in *A Directory of Self-Help/Mutual Aid Support Groups for Older People with Impaired Vision.*[13] An additional guide for information about state services/sponsorship is the *Directory of Services for Blind and Visually Impaired Persons in the United States and Canada.*[1]

Low vision billing should conform to the standards of good practice the office maintains in billing for other services. Just as with other billing, it is important to establish a clear audit trail and to monitor claim payments.

Because of the variety of services and providers in low vision care and the limitations of existing reimbursement plans, it is not unusual for a combination of payment sources to be approached for an individual patient. The practice's ability to access multiple reimbursement sources is beneficial to the patient (and to the practice) because it can minimize out-of-pocket expense. However, it can be confusing to staff, and difficult to handle completely by electronic billing. Patients, too, may find it difficult to understand the limitations of different programs. Only you can weigh the advantages and disadvantages of making multiple reimbursement sources available to your patients.

Adapting Your Office Suite

CLINICAL PEARL

Adapting the examination room and the instruction area include provision for special equipment, charts, and devices for testing and demonstration to patients, task lighting, and products for daily living activities.

The Examination Room

In addition to the basic diagnostic equipment, the low vision examination room should have a set of full diameter, loose trial lenses, prism lenses, and a trial frame. Acuity charts for distance and near in logMAR[14] notation, and a continuous text reading card with graduated print size should be included. Function tests including Amsler grid, a contrast sensitivity test, and brightness acuity test are necessary along with color identification material such as paint chips, the Holmgren wool test, or the Quantitative Color Vision Test. A basic set of low vision devices should include spectacles, hand and stand magnifiers of comparable strengths, telescopes, absorptive lenses, and nonoptical devices. (See the list of suggested equipment later in the chapter.) A videomagnifier may be made available in the office, or other arrangements made to demonstrate it to patients as needed.

All lenses should be labeled by strength and manufacturer/catalogue number to reduce prescribing and reordering difficulties. If you will have multiple examination rooms with like equipment, color coding the devices by room is very helpful. A cabinet containing four to five trays, drawers, or shelves will be needed to hold the optical equipment.

The Instruction Area

A separate space should be allocated for instruction. If possible, a separate room is ideal because it frees the examination room and helps the person with low vision to make the transition from being a patient to being a learner during the instruction phase of the examination.

The work station in the instruction area will need a nonglare tabletop and chairs for the instructor, the patient, and the friend or family member. There should be ample outlets at table height so that illuminated devices can be demonstrated easily. Include a variety of styles of task lighting and bulbs in different wattages. Other supplies include local newspapers (and foreign language papers if necessary), large print books, religious reading material, bank statements, utility bills, labels, needlework supplies, and a reading stand. Other consumer products for activities of daily living (such as large-number timers, address books, watches, digital thermometers, "talking" calculators, self-threading needles), and catalogues showing these products, are also helpful.[15] Having referral and resource material available allows you to make a timely connection for the patient to services you do not offer. The equipment in the lending system (if there is one) may be stored in the instruction room or in the dispensing area. Take-home information for patients is useful to have in the instruction area including pamphlets, device use/care instructions, catalogues, applications for other services/benefits, and descriptions of local services/organizations.

CLINICAL PEARL

Having referral and resource material available allows you to make a timely connection for the patient to services you do not offer.

Dispensing

Planning how, where, and when the patient is going to obtain the optical and adaptive devices is a critical piece of the service delivery package. Dispensing from the office has advantages for the clinician and the patient, but requires planning to implement. Setting up a low vision dispensing unit within the practice requires the allocation of space, the purchase of a supply of devices for resale, staff training, and pricing. The basic supply of devices can parallel the selected diagnostic low vision equipment.

CLINICAL PEARL

Planning how, where, and when the patient is going to obtain the optical and adaptive devices is a critical piece of the service delivery package.

Some practices dispense the low vision devices directly from their diagnostic equipment supply. While this seems like a cost effective approach, it can interfere with the lenses available for other examinations, and it clouds the distinction between depreciable equipment and resale items. Another strategy (for practices that incorporate the use of a "loaner" device in their low vision services) is to loan *new* items and allow the patient to buy the loaned lens (rather than maintaining a loan inventory that circulates to many patients). This approach can also help to build a loan system slowly, as items which may be rejected by patients during the loan period are returned to become part of a circulating inventory.

Using a community optician to sell devices you prescribe is another alternative but requires careful coordination. The optician should stock a supply of devices that parallels your diagnostic low vision devices, and should receive training in how to reinforce correct device use techniques. With this approach, communication is very important. The optician will have information about the patient's acceptance of the device and, just as with routine eyeglass prescriptions, should report results and problems to you.

Choosing Equipment for the Practice

For years The Lighthouse, through its continuing education program in low vision, has consulted both with practitioners who are introducing low vision care into their practices and with those who are planning to offer more extensive care. The considerations and suggestions that follow are based on the results of these consultations and reflect the core of low vision practice. Each practice is different. Additional devices should be added to the core based on your patient profile (eye disease, vision, age, work/leisure, etc.), practice location, your training, and the extent of services you offer. Cost information is offered as a guideline only, and of course is subject to change.[16]

CLINICAL PEARL

Each practice is different. Additional devices should be added to the core based on your patient profile (eye disease, vision, age, work/leisure, etc.), practice location, your training, and the extent of services you offer.

Acuity and Function Tests

Specialized visual acuity and function tests are necessary in order to deliver low vision care. Many practices already may have some or all of this testing material used diagnostically for their regular patients.
- Acuity charts (distance and near) - $150 to $250
- Contrast charts - $450 to $500

- Brightness acuity test (BAT) - $800
- Color test - $75 to $300
- Amsler grid manual - $75
- Chart illuminator and stand - $825

Diagnostic Optical Equipment

The following devices are recommended for low vision practice.

Spectacles and Loupes

What to consider when choosing spectacles and loupes:
- You will need base-in prisms, and a range of aspheric, high-plus lenses in two diopter increments. For testing, have glasses made up OU.
- Choose a variety of frame colors that do not draw attention to the eyewear.
- Have strength engraved on temples.
- For the diagnostic set the average frame size is 44/22 with 140 mm temples.

Spectacle types and dioptric power:
- Base-in prism spectacles in full or half frames come in +4 to +12 with appropriate prism.
    Usual selection: +6, +8, +10
    Approximate total cost for usual selection:
    $150 (high index $400)
- Aspheric Lenticular Full Frame Spectacles come in +10 to +20
    Usual selection: +10, +12, +16, +20
    Approximate total cost for usual selection: $180
- Aspheric Lenticular Microscopic Full or Half Frame spectacles come in + 24 (6X), to +48 (12X)
    Usual selection: +24 (6X), +32 (8X)
    Approximate total cost for usual selection: $100 (half frame); $160 (full frame)
- Doublets, available with high index glass and anti-reflection coating, come in 2X (8D) to 8X (32 D)
    Usual selection: 6X, 7X, 8X
    Approximate total cost for usual selection:
    $145 each eye, $275 OU

Loupe types and dioptric power:
- Headborne or clip-on, monocular and binocular come in +2 to +32
    Usual selection: 6D (2.5X), 10D (3.5X), 15D (4.75X)
    Approximate total cost for usual selection: $70

Hand magnifiers

What to consider when choosing hand magnifiers:
- Represent a range of costs.
- Have samples from many manufacturers.
- Choose a variety of strengths.

- Patients prefer rectangular magnifiers to round ones.
- Illuminated magnifiers are good for shopping and restaurants. However, batteries are expensive and bulbs and batteries are often difficult for arthritic hands to manage.
- Know that hand magnifiers mounted on an arm or in a clamp are useful for specific tasks.

Types and dioptric power: illuminated and nonilluminated come in +5 to +68

Usual selection: +5 to +48 (12X)

Approximate total cost for usual selection: $600

Stand magnifiers

What to consider when choosing stand magnifiers:
- Represent a range of costs.
- Choose strengths that cover the range of powers available.
- Having some illuminated stand magnifiers is essential.

Types and dioptric power: illuminated and nonilluminated +2 to +88

Usual selection: +3.5 to +60

Approximate total cost for usual selection: $600

Telescopes

What to consider when choosing telescopes:
- Represent a range of powers in various styles and types.
- Select distance and near telescopes.
- Some handheld telescopes can be adapted to spectacle-mount.

Types and magnification: handheld, clip-on, spectacle-mounted; 1.7X to 10X

Usual selection: 2X to 6X

Approximate total cost for usual selection: $220 to $1500 (single telescopes or diagnostic kits)

Absorptive lenses

What to consider when choosing absorptive lenses:
- Represent a variety of colors and frame styles.
- Consider storing absorptive lenses in an easy-to-carry box or case to facilitate trial outdoors (or at a window).

Types: fixed and variable transmittance, clip-on, fit-over, instant (behind lens), flip-up, nonprescription and prescription

Usual selection: greys, plums, yellows, ambers variety of types, luminous transmittance from 90% to 1%, UV absorption at or above 400 nm

Approximate total cost for usual selection: $200 to $400

Electronic magnifiers

Closed circuit television reading systems, computer programs that produce large print and voice output, are available. These systems provide an excellent alternative for the person who requires greater working distance, has severely impaired vision, and/or needs to use a computer in school, on the job, or for personal business. Before you make a decision to have a particular electronic system available in your office, you may want to arrange for a demonstration by the sales representative and a discussion of sales/loan arrangements. You may also want to inquire whether a system is available for your patients to see in your local library or school system, or vision rehabilitation agency.

Nonoptical devices

Nonoptical devices are important vision aids and consist of large print or enlarged type books, newspapers, and periodicals; other enlarged print devices such as calculators, clocks, watches, timers, thermostats, games, playing cards, bold-ruled paper, and felt-tipped pens; and medical devices such as digital thermometers, insulin guides, and scales. You will need to have a sample of the equipment operating instruction and you may want samples of some of the products in your office. You should also have resource information available so patients will know how to obtain these items.

Adaptive and accessory devices

Adaptive devices such as reading stands and lap desks can be used alone or in conjunction with optical devices. Accessory devices include typoscopes, signature guides, acetate overlays, clamps, and other products to enhance daily living.

Lamps and lighting

These include lamps with an adjustable arm and reflectors to focus the light directly on the task and reduce heat, lamps that incorporate magnifiers (magnification is usually from +1.7 to +10), flashlights (halogen, mobility flashlight, and miniature focusable), and bulbs—indoor reflector, neodymium, yellow tint (bug light), and soft white.

Optical device lending system

Many clinicians use a lending system where the person may take lenses home for a practice and reinforcement period of up to 2 weeks following examination and instruction. Incorporating a lending system relieves the pressure of immediate choice in the test environment and improves the success rate. Data from The Lighthouse Inc. Low Vision Services indicate that 45% of patients borrow a lens.

The devices in a lending system frequently parallel the diagnostic equipment with a few exceptions. Not available for loan are inexpensive devices and absorptive lenses. Other supplies necessary to maintain a lending system are disposable plastic bags in which to send equipment home, extra frames, and a logging system to keep track of items due for return. If you use a device lending system, remember to build time into the schedule for instructors to talk with patients during the loan/practice period. Through this contact the instructor can reinforce proper device usage, identify device-use problems, and adjust the loaner period if the patient is having extreme difficulties.

Other equipment

It is also useful to have inexpensive, portable amplifying devices in the office when examining a person who has a hearing impairment.

Referral and Resource Information for Vision Rehabilitation

A recent survey shows that many middle-aged and older Americans are not aware of the vision rehabilitation resources available to them.[17] For the practice with a commitment to comprehensive low vision care—regardless of the level of service provided within the practice— informing the patient about these services, and making timely referrals, should be viewed as a routine step in the care that is given. Understanding that specialized rehabilitation/counseling services are available through state and private vision rehabilitation agencies and hospitals and knowing their referral criteria; and maintaining other resources such as lists of community services, catalogues of consumer products, pamphlets on eye disease and low vision, and advocacy and self-help groups is essential to low vision practice. This information is easily obtainable from local and national sources. You can help to "complete the loop" for your patients by providing them with the referrals and resources necessary to complete their vision rehabilitation.

CLINICAL PEARL

For the practice with a commitment to comprehensive low vision care— regardless of the level of service provided within the practice—informing the patient about these services, and making timely referrals, should be viewed as a routine step in the care that is given.

References

1. American Foundation for the Blind: *Directory of services for blind and visually impaired persons in the United States and Canada,* ed 24, New York, 1993, American Foundation for the Blind.
2. National Center for Health Statistics: Advance data from vital and health statistics, No 125, DHHS Pub. No. (PHS) 86-1250, Public health Service, Hyattsville, Md, 1986, National Center for Health Statistics.
3. National Center for Health Statistics. Havlik RJ: *Aging in the eighties, impaired senses for sound and light in persons age 65 years and over,* Preliminary data from the Supplement on Aging to the National Health Interview Survey, United States, Jan-June 1984.

4. Offner R: *ADA accessibility guidelines: provisions for people with impaired vision*, New York, 1994, The Lighthouse Inc.
5. Knoblauch K, Arditi A: *Designing effective color contrast for the partially sighted*, Technical Report VR02, New York, 1993, The Lighthouse Inc.
6. The Lighthouse Inc: Examination form for low vision available by written request to Lighthouse Continuing Education, 111 East 59th Street, New York, NY 10022
7. Freeman P, Jose R: *The art and practice of low vision*, Boston, 1991, Butterworth-Heinemann.
8. The Lighthouse Inc: *Print legibility and partial sight*, New York, 1994, The Lighthouse Inc.
9. The Lighthouse Inc: *Lighthouse continuing education course catalog 1995-96*, New York, The Lighthouse Inc.
10. Fletcher D, Weinstock F: How to use CPT codes for low vision rehabilitation, *ARGUS* January 1991, p. 13.
11. American Medical Association: *Physicians' current procedural terminology*, Chicago, 1995, American Medical Association.
12. Practice Management Information Corp: *International classification of diseases, 9th revision*, ed 3, Los Angeles, 1989, Practice Management Information Corp.
13. The Lighthouse Inc: *Self-help/mutual aid support groups for visually impaired older people: a guide and directory*, ed 2, New York, 1994, The Lighthouse Inc.
14. Johnson A: Making sense of the M, N and logMAR systems of specifying visual acuity. In: *Problems in optometry*, Philadelphia, 1991, JB Lippencott, 394-407.
15. The Lighthouse Inc: *Consumer products catalog*, New York, 1994-95, The Lighthouse Inc.
16. The Lighthouse Inc: *Lighthouse low vision products catalog for professionals*, ed 8, New York, 1994, The Lighthouse Inc.
17. The Lighthouse Inc: *The lighthouse national survey on vision loss: the experiences, attitudes and knowledge of middle aged and older Americans*, New York, 1995, The Lighthouse Inc.

13

A Functional Approach to the Fitting of Spectacle-Mounted Telescopic Systems

Bruce P. Rosenthal
Wayne W. Hoeft

Key Terms

Galilean telescope	exit pupil	bioptic
Keplerian telescope	pupillary distance	

The importance of interpupillary measurement in the fitting of telescopic systems for the visually impaired was first described by Bruner[1] in 1930, when he simply stated, "Great care must be taken in making all frame measurements." Shortly thereafter Feinbloom[2] wrote an introduction to *The Principles and Practice of Sub-Normal Vision Correction* in which he noted that the first specification, for Telescopes or Microscopes, should include the pupillary distance. . . "When the finished glasses are returned from the manufacturer, they should be checked for alignment. If the telescopes are properly aligned, only one target will be visible. That is, the image in each eye will be fused. If they are not properly aligned, two images will be seen." It is therefore apparent that the difficulties in interpupillary measurement were recognized early on, especially in preventing a common complaint of diplopia.

Fitting the Microspiral Galilean Telescope[3]

The microspiral Galilean telescopes, which are also known as the Clear View I and II lenses, are miniature Galilean focusable telescopes that were designed for cosmetic appearance as well as being light-weight. They have a focal range from 25 cm to infinity.

One of the distinct disadvantages of the Clear View I (Figure 13-1), which ranged in powers of 2.2X, 2.7X, 3.3X, 4X, 5X and 6X, was the 9 mm diameter of the lens. But the chief difficulty in the fitting was matching the minute exit pupil of the telescope (Figure 13-2) with the entrance pupil of the eye. Another objection by patients was that the size of the field, which ranged in size from 7.0 degrees for the 2.2X to 3 degrees for the 6.0X, was difficult to fit and align. To counteract the difficulty of fitting the Clear View I, Hoeft designed a fitting frame (Figure 13-3) in which the 2.2X through the 6.0X could be fitted either monocularly or binocularly.

Once the telescope is placed in the fitting frame, a transilluminator is directed through the telescope to the pupil. The transilluminator gives a better spot of light than a penlight. The system generally aligns quite rapidly using this method. Hoeft suggests that the clinician prefocus the telescope before handing it to the patient, and that the lenses being fit in the bioptic position be positioned 6 to 9 mm above the pupil.

CLINICAL PEARL

Hoeft suggests that the clinician prefocus the telescope before handing it to the patient.

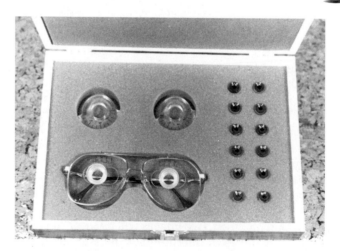

FIGURE 13-1 Clear View I fitting set.

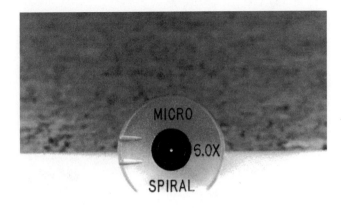

FIGURE 13-2 Exit pupil of microspiral telescope. Note the minute size of the exit pupil in the center of the picture.

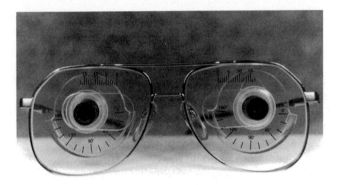

FIGURE 13-3 Hoeft fitting frame.

A New Fitting Frame for Galilean and Spectacle-Mounted Telescopic Systems

At a time when Hoeft was working on the microspiral fitting system, Rosenthal was designing a frame, similar in concept to the Hoeft design, that would accommodate the Designs for Vision fixed focus 3.0X Galilean telescope. This fitting system was reminiscent of the Polysnap design[4] which was developed by Rosenthal and Freed in the late 1970s. The Polysnap was an industrial frame with polycarbonate lenses which accommodated the 2.5X and 2.8X Galilean Selsi telescopes

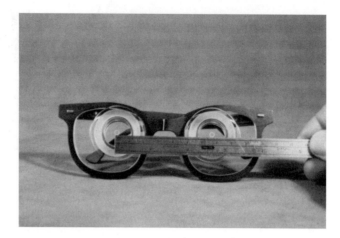

FIGURE 13-4 Yeoman fitting frame. Note the line in the center of the bridge for measuring monocular PDs.

and the 4.0×12 Keplerian design. Fitting was often a problem with the Polysnap frame. Polysnap systems, especially when the telescopic system was heavy (e.g., 4×12, 6×16), tended to "tip" on the patient's face, thereby causing alignment problems with the patient's visual axis and the optical axis of the system. The Polysnap again illustrated the fitting problems that occurred when the exit pupil of the telescope was not exactly aligned with the entrance pupil of the eye. Another drawback of the Polysnap was the inability to fit the system binocularly. Binocular systems were virtually impossible to fit because there was no mechanism for exact collimation.

Rosenthal modified his fitting frame design to accommodate the Galilean as well as Keplerian telescopes (Figure 13-4). The fitting frames have a rectangular cutout to accurately determine the monocular pupillary distance. A fitting set was also designed with a pair of focusable Galilean telescopes ranging in power from 2.2X to 4.0X, and pairs of Keplerian telescopes ranging in power from 2.0X to 6.0X. The set also includes an occluder that can be placed over one eye to accurately determine the appropriate monocular magnification that satisfies the patient's objectives. In fact the clinician can rapidly insert a Galilean telescope or Keplerian telescope of the same power to compare the field, weight, and cosmetic appearance of each system.

CLINICAL PEARL

Rosenthal modified his fitting frame design to accommodate the Galilean as well as Keplerian telescopes.

Pupillary distance can be accurately determined by monocularly sliding the aperture until the visual axis is centered through the opening. A small plastic disc with a pinhole pupil can be centered over the visual axis and confirmed with a transilluminator. The telescope can then be inserted and the patient should be able to see the object of regard with little frustration. The advantages of this fitting system are as follows:

1. The patient can see the actual telescopic system that will be prescribed.
2. Galilean telescopes as well as Keplerian telescopes can be fit in the same frame. (Figure 13-5)
3. Galilean and Keplerian telescopes can be compared for weight, cosmetics, field of view, and light gathering ability.
4. The heavy trial frame can be eliminated.
5. The patient's prescription can be incorporated in the rear cell with an adapting clip.
6. It only takes a few minutes to test the type and power of spectacle-mounted telescopes that are used by 95% of the low vision patients.
7. This fitting system can also accommodate the microspiral II Galilean telescopes (Figure 13-6).

The technique developed by Rosenthal is as follows:

1. Select the appropriate size Yeoman frame from the fitting set (e.g., 46/22/6) (Fig. 13-4).
2. Determine the pupillary distance by moving the slot to center the visual axis with the opening. Use the plastic cap with the pinhole opening and a transilluminator if necessary.
3. Insert the telescopes, whether Galilean or Keplerian (Fig. 13-5).

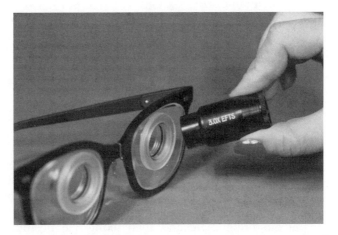

FIGURE 13-5 Keplerian telescope being inserted into the Designs for Vision Yeoman fitting frame.

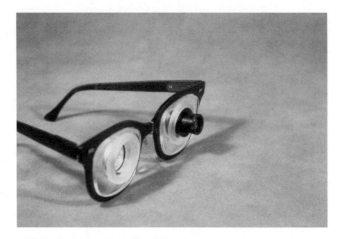

FIGURE 13-6 Yeoman fitting frame from the BATMAN trial set of Keplerian and Galilean telescopic fitting set that is modified to accept the microspiral II Galilean telescope.

    4. Order the final telescope with the following in mind:
       a. Carrier correction
       b. Type of system/Galilean or Keplerian/monocular/binocular
       c. Telescopic position
          i. Bioptic
         ii. Full diameter
        iii. This is not intended as a reading (surgical) fitting system–the Englemann technique is recommended for determining the near pupillary distance.
       d. System correction
       e. Frame size

Fitting the Ocutech Vision Enhancing System[5]

Greene developed the Keplerian Ocutech Vision Enhancing System (VES) to address the need for a wider field of view and greater magnification. The VES, which combines a periscope (Horizontal Light Path Enhancing System HLP-VES) and Keplerian telescope into one design, lies across the top of the eyeglass lens rather than extending forward out from the front of the eyeglass lens.

The HLP-VES (Figure 13-7) is completely adjustable for all fitting controls so that no preliminary measurements are required. Pupillary distance is adjusted by sliding the telescope to the right or the left on the mounting plate and then fixing the position with set screws (Figure 13-8). The angle of inclination of the telescope and the vertex distance can be controlled by loosening screws at each end of the

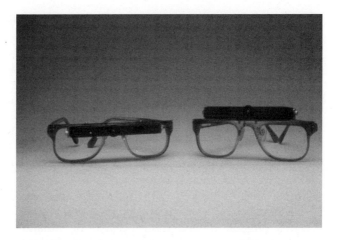

FIGURE 13-7 HLP-VES in upper and lower position.

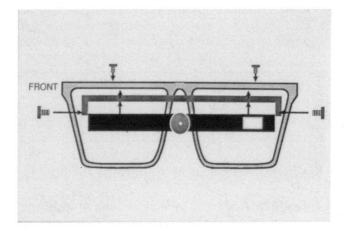

FIGURE 13-8 Set screws on the Ocutech HLP-VES system to adjust for interpupillary distance and angle of the telescope.

telescope through the mounting bracket. In addition, by removing these two end screws, the telescope can be removed from the bracket and flipped over to be positioned for use by either the right or the left eye. The telescope can be mounted in either the standard, above the frame position or, by using an alternate mounting bracket, can be positioned in a lower full-diameter position for intermediate and near applications.

Only the specially designed frame can be used with the HLP-VES (Figure 13-7). It is designed to position low on the bridge, resembling a half eye frame, with a flat plate across the top to accept the telescope mounting bracket. The frame provides a wide range of fitting control by way of adjustable bridge guard arms, and two adult front sizes and temple lengths. A pediatric-size frame is also available. The frame is deep enough to allow for multifocal fitting; however, because the frame is intended to sit low on the bridge, segments are fit higher than normal, and the optical center should be positioned approximately 10 mm higher than the geometric center of the frame. An alternate style frame is available that allows for telescope mounting when carrier lens prescriptions are not desired.

Greene notes that as with all telescopic systems, fitting the telescope as close to the eye as possible increases the field of view through the HLP-VES. The side screws allow for sliding the telescope forward or backward to position it as closely as possible. Of great importance, especially with the Keplerian telescopes, is the precise positioning of the exit pupil along the line of sight. This positioning is often difficult to determine because of variations in angle kappa, eccentric viewing, and nystagmus. A slight misalignment may still provide a full field through the telescope but may reduce overall retinal illumination, decreasing perceived image brightness. By allowing the patient to slide the telescope right and left to achieve a full and bright image, accurate alignment can be readily achieved.

CLINICAL PEARL

Greene notes that as with all telescopic systems, fitting the telescope as close to the eye as possible increases the field of view through the HLP-VES.

Fitting the Bi-Telemicroscopic Apparatus (BITA) [6]

The BITA is another miniature Galilean telescope that has a unique patented bi-level positioning system that is mounted in a shaded lens (Figure 13-9). The BITA is positioned and angled in the patient's carrier lens in such a manner that while looking straight ahead, the wearer's line of sight is just below the miniature telescope. This alignment of the telescopic axis with the patient's line of sight is termed the bi-level or simulvision mounting position. The bi-level feature allows for both a magnified and unmagnified view of the object of regard simultaneously. In the patient's visual field, these views are so close that they touch or adjoin. The proximity of the two views allows the perception of an object in the field without loss of perspective given by the unmagnified perception.

CLINICAL PEARL

The bi-level feature allows for both a magnified and unmagnified view of the object of regard simultaneously.

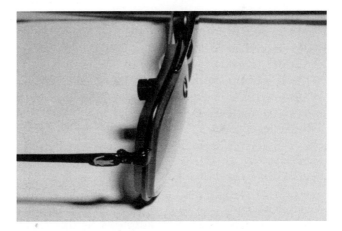

FIGURE 13-9 BITA system with tinted carrier lens.

Williams suggests placing a 2.5× or a 3.0× BITA unit of either $\frac{5}{16}$ or $\frac{3}{8}$ inch diameter before the better eye. The units can be placed into a trial frame, or a special frame from Eschenbach with adaptor rings, or the units may be handheld. The position of the BITA is determined from the position of the line of sight. The fitting manual describes a series of different methods to determine the positioning of the line of sight position while the patient is fixing on a distant object. One method involves the use of a small piece of adhesive tape that contains a small hole approximately $\frac{1}{8}$ inch in diameter. The tape is fixed to the carrier lenses and is moved until the line of sight is fixed on a distant object through the hole. If binocular units are being prescribed, the patient should perceive a single hole in the binocular mode.

To achieve the bi-level effect, the laboratory will calculate the exact position to drill the scopes based on the location of the line of sight. Another method involves the use of small colored filter dots attached to the carrier lenses. With this method, the filter dots are moistened and affixed to the carriers and moved into the line of sight while the patient is fixating a distant object. Small adjustments to the temples and pantoscopic angle of the frame will locate the position of the dot to determine the line of sight position. Williams suggests repeating the measurements a few times to ensure consistency.

When the BITA is prescribed for reading, the units will necessarily be directed in a downward position. With the diameter of the unit and the power having already been determined for best response, the location of the telescope is based on the patient's functional IPD (interpupillary distance) at the desired reading distance. The laboratory will drill the carrier for the correct convergence and angling according to the diameter of the unit, the functional IPD, and the working distance desired. To determine how much the frame is angled in reference to the true perpendicular of the ground, and to determine the angle at which to drill the carrier lenses, a reading is made with a device called the perpendicular reference indicator (PRI). This device, similar to a protractor, is attached to the right temple and a reading is made indicating the amount of head tilt in the straight ahead viewing position. With this measurement the technician can then align the machinery to duplicate the position and drill the hole to accommodate the BITA unit at the correct position to accomplish the bi-level effect.

Fitting the Behind-the-Lens Telescope[7]

Spitzberg, Jose, and Kuether described the behind-the-lens telescope as a telescopic system that provides the advantage of improved cosmetics with its miniaturized design and placement behind the spectacle lens, as well as having Keplerian optics (Figure 13-10) for a wide field of view. The original placement of the system was behind the spectacle carrier lens in an inferior or inferior temporal position. The objective lens was flush with the front surface of the carrier lens with the added advantage of being able to place a clip-on filter over the spectacle lens, making the telescope essentially invisible to the eye.

Spitzberg et al. recommended that to achieve clinical success the practitioner should first show the patient the mock-up frame/ telescope and explain that the telescope fits inferiorly behind the spectacle. The system is arranged so that the patient looks inferiorly through the telescope to see what is straight ahead or in the direction the nose is pointing. The nose can be a reference point for initial localization. Without this reference of looking straight ahead at what

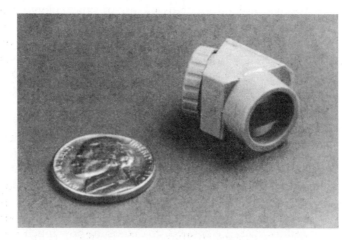

FIGURE 13-10 Keplerian optics for the behind-the-lens telescope.

they want to see and looking through the telescope, patients can have difficulty localizing through the system, even when the clinician has it aligned. At first patients may want to move their head.

CLINICAL PEARL

Spitzberg et al. recommended that to achieve clinical success the practitioner should first show the patient the mock-up frame/telescope.

Spitzberg recommends the following for the new inferior position (Figure 13-11):

1. Adjust the demo frame on the patient making sure it has a *flat face form* and *no* pantoscopic tilt. (It already comes to the examiner that way.)
2. Place the telescope in the carrier lens before the better eye. Make sure you have the telescope focused for the test distance. (You may want to mark this point on the ocular. It should already be marked for distance for an emmetrope.)
3. Place the frame on the patient. The horizontal line on the lens should be approximately at the pupil center height. Adjust the nosepads to move the frame up and down until this position is reached.

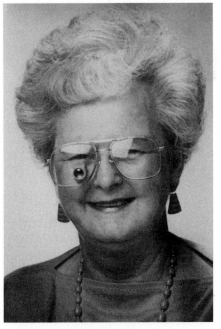

FIGURE 13-11 Behind-the-lens telescope in the inferior position. (Photo courtesy of Dr. Larry Spitzberg.)

4. Set the telescope in the carrier straight up and down. This approximates a 62 PD. For smaller PDs turn the telescope inward; for larger PDs turn the telescope outward.
5. Have the patient look at or point the nose at the distance chart. Then have the patient look down (35 degrees) into the telescope without moving the head. (You may suggest it works like looking into a bifocal.)
6. The patient should see the chart. (If not, the patient may have moved the head downward and may be looking at the floor, or the frame may be adjusted incorrectly.)

References

1. Bruner AB: Telescopic lenses as an aid to poor vision, *Am Ophthalmol* vol. 2, September, 1929, 668.
2. Feinbloom W: Report of 500 cases of sub-normal vision, *Am J Optom Arch Am Acad Optom,* vol 8, 1933, 122, 238.
3. Hoeft WW: *The microspiral Galilean telescope in a structured approach to low vision care.* Ed. Rosenthal and Cole, vol 3, Lippincott, No. 3, Philadelphia, 1991, 490-94.
4. Rosenthal BP: *Fitting spectacle telescopes and glasses in clinical low vision.* Ed. Faye EE, Boston, 1984, Little, Brown & Co, 149.
5. Green HA: The ocutech vision enhancing system (VES) a new low vision spectacle telescopic system. In Rosenthal BP, Cole RG (eds): *A structured approach to low vision care,* Lippincott, vol 3, no. 3, Philadelphia, 1991, 484-489.
6. Williams DR: The bi-level telemicroscopic apparatus - (BITA). In Rosenthal BP, Cole RG (eds): *A structured approach to low vision care,* Lippincott, vol 3, No. 3, 1991, 495-503.
7. Spitzburg LA, Jose RT, Kuether CL: The behind-the-lens telescope. In Rosenthal BP, Cole RG (eds): *A structured approach to low vision care,* Lippincott, vol 3, No. 3, Philadelphia, 1991, 504-509.

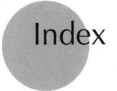

Index

Page numbers in *italic type* refer to figures. Tables are indicated by *t* following the page number.

A

Aberrations
  in aspheric curve lenses, 186
  in CR-39 lenses, 183
  in high index lenses, 184
  in polycarbonate lenses, 185
Absorptive lenses, for low vision practices, 262
Accessory contrast control devices, 79-92
Accidents, automobile, visual attention and, 229-230
Accommodation assessments, for visual efficiency training, 4-65
Achromatopsia, 81
Acuity predictions, eccentric viewing and, 35-36
ADA; *see* Americans with Disabilities Act (ADA)
Adaptive devices, 71-121
  dispensing of, 259-260
  lighting controls for, 79-92
  for low vision practices, 263
  for medical assistance, 99-103
  mobility assistive, 103-112
  for posture and positioning, 92-97
  relative size, 72-79
  for sensory substitution, 112-119

Adaptive devices—cont'd
  for writing and communication, 97-99
Add power, 140
Add-on boards, for computer access programs, 205
Adnexa, anti-infective drugs for, 128
Adrenergic agonist drugs
  adverse ocular effects of, 131
  decongestants, 127
  for lowering intraocular pressure, 131
  mydriatics, 125-126
Afocal telescopes
  optical principles of, 160-164, *163*
  with/without reading caps, 165, *165*
Allergic conjunctivitis, seasonal treatment of, 126-127
Allergic rhinitis, antihistamines for, 133
Americans with Disabilities Act (ADA), 198-199
  typography and, 247
Ametropic patients, telescopes for, 161, 162
Aminoketone antidepressants, adverse systemic effects of, 135*t*

M

Optometric Extension Program
(OEP), 65
Overall visual field loss
enhancement techniques, 23-24
Fresnel prisms for, 20-21,
22-23, *23*
minification for, 17-19, *18*
minus lens minifiers for, 20-21, *21*
reverse telescopes for, 19-20
treatment of, 16-24

P

Paper, adaptive devices for,
98-99, *99*
Paperless braille, 118
Paroxetine, adverse systemic effects
of, 135*t*
Partial prisms
clinical management of, 14-15
for hemianopia, 12-15, *13, 14*
Pastpointing
eccentric fixation and, 35
testing for, 35
Pathsounders, 107-108
Patient assessments
computer access sophistication,
204
distance spectacles and, 180
for eccentric viewing, 30-38
of pharmaceutical effects, 123-137
for visual efficiency training,
61-63, 62*t*
for visual rehabilitation training,
61-63
Pegboard rotators, for eccentric
viewing
training, 46, *46*
Pens, for visually impaired, 98-99
Pepper Visual Skills Analysis Test, 63
Perceived magnification, 168
Perceptual assessments, for visual
efficiency training, 65
Perceptual filling, blind spot
awareness and, 40
Personal computers, computer access
programs and, large print, *204*

Pharmaceuticals; *see* specific kinds of
drugs, e.g., Paroxetine
Phenethylamine antidepressants,
adverse systemic effects of, 135*t*
Pheniramine maleate, 127
Phenylephrine, 127
for diagnostic evaluation, 125-126
for pupil dilation, 125-126
for visual field testing in
glaucoma, 126
Photochromic lenses, 194
Photophobia, 80-81
Pleioptic training, for eccentric
viewing, 43
Pleioptics, visual field testing and, 37
PLS filters; *see* Younger Protective
Lens Series (PLS) filters
Polycarbonate lenses
for distance spectacles, 181,
184, 185
filters and, 194
Postchiasmal neurological insult, 2
Post-training assessments, visual
efficiency training and, 67-68
Posture and positioning devices,
92-97
in design of hand magnifiers,
96, *97*
Posture Rite Lap Desks, 94, *96*
for reading, 92-95, *93, 94, 95*
for telescopic devices, 96-97, *97*
Posture Rite Lap Desks, 94, *96*
Preferred retinal locus (PRL), 29-30
scanning laser ophthalmoscopes
and, 36-37
visual field tests and, 37
Prismatic displacement, for eccentric
viewing training, 39-40
Prisms, *8*
clinical management of, 22-23
Fresnel, 10, 12-13, 15, 22-23, *23*
for computer monitors, 201
full field, *9*, 9-12
clinical management of, 11-12
ground-in, 10
for hemianopia, 7-15
for overall visual field loss, 22-23